Clinical Challenges
& Images in
GASTROENTEROLOGY

A Diagnostic Guide

Siew C Ng

Heyson CH Chan

Rashid NS Lui

tfm Publishing Limited, Castle Hill Barns, Harley, Shrewsbury, SY5 6LX, UK
Tel: +44 (0)1952 510061; Fax: +44 (0)1952 510192
E-mail: info@tfmpublishing.com
Web site: www.tfmpublishing.com

Editing, design & typesetting: Nikki Bramhill BSc Hons Dip Law

First edition: © 2018
Paperback   ISBN: 978-1-910079-03-4

E-book editions: 2018
ePub   ISBN: 978-1-910079-04-1
Mobi   ISBN: 978-1-910079-05-8
Web pdf   ISBN: 978-1-910079-06-5

Printed by Gutenberg Press Ltd., Gudja Road, Tarxien, Malta, GXQ 2902
Tel: +356 218 97037; Fax: +356 218 00069
E-mail: info@gutenberg.com.mt
Web site: www.gutenberg.com.mt

Contents

Contents

Preface

Digestive diseases have always been a major threat to global health. Despite the rapid advances in various diagnostic modalities, many a time the final verdict can be elusive and present a diagnostic challenge for the attending doctor. "Clinical Challenges & Images in Gastroenterology — A Diagnostic Guide" presents 45 real-life cases to illustrate an evidence-based approach to the diagnosis, investigation and management of gastrointestinal diseases commonly encountered in everyday practice, with a special focus on the interpretation of endoscopic and radiological images. This book provides a pragmatic approach for medical students, residents, specialist trainees and specialists alike who have an interest in gastroenterology and hepatology. Other healthcare providers, such as general practitioners, nurses and dieticians, will also benefit from these case illustrations.

A unique feature of this book is that virtually all of the cases were managed by a multi-disciplinary team at the Prince of Wales Hospital, Hong Kong. The Editors of this book are based at the Institute of Digestive Disease, The Chinese University of Hong Kong. Our Institute founded by Professor Joseph Sung a decade ago has contributed to major breakthroughs that have improved the clinical management of digestive diseases including, but not limited to, the advent of advanced endoscopic therapies and minimally invasive surgery, molecular diagnostic tools for cancers and inflammatory bowel disease, and the development of novel treatments for acid peptic disease and viral hepatitis. The past directors of our Institute, Professor Francis Chan and Professor Henry Chan, are leaders in the fields of gastroenterology and hepatology.

This book aims to promote integrative and interdisciplinary medicine in digestive diseases. Our vision was to provide a variety of GI cases accompanied by diagnostic and management approaches to achieve the best outcomes for patients in day-to-day practice. Key take home messages for each case are highlighted under the sections of "Clinical pearls" and "Impress your attending".

We were fortunate to have received excellent training in the United Kingdom and Hong Kong. The opportunity to work together on this book was a unique one — an idea that was developed during weekly GI rounds. We not only enjoy each other's stimulating ideas, but also share the same passion in advancing and pioneering practice for GI diseases.

Our thanks go to Dr. Raymond Tang (Institute of Digestive Disease), Professor Anthony Chan and Dr. Maribel Lacambra (Department of Anatomical and Cellular Pathology), Dr. Esther Hung and Dr. Eric Law (Department of Imaging and Interventional Radiology) for providing important pathology and imaging input. We are also grateful to our fellow gastroenterologists, Dr. Joyce Mak and Professor Sunny Wong, for providing valuable comments on the cases.

Importantly, this endeavour would not have been possible without our publisher, Nikki Bramhill (Director, tfm publishing Ltd). It has been a real pleasure and delight to work with Nikki. Her energy, efficiency and vision to transfer knowledge in the most effective way have allowed this partnership to flourish with much happiness.

Siew C Ng MBBS (UK), FRCP (Lond, Edin), PhD (Lond), AGAF, FHKCP, FHKAM (Medicine)
Professor and Honorary Consultant
Institute of Digestive Disease
Department of Medicine and Therapeutics
Prince of Wales Hospital, The Chinese University of Hong Kong

Heyson CH Chan MBChB (CUHK), MRCP (UK), FHKCP, FHKAM (Medicine)
Associate Consultant and Honorary Clinical Assistant Professor
Institute of Digestive Disease
Department of Medicine and Therapeutics
Prince of Wales Hospital, The Chinese University of Hong Kong

Rashid NS Lui MBChB (CUHK), MRCP (UK), FHKCP, FHKAM (Medicine)
Resident Specialist and Honorary Clinical Tutor
Institute of Digestive Disease
Department of Medicine and Therapeutics
Prince of Wales Hospital, The Chinese University of Hong Kong

Abbreviations

AAA	Abdominal aortic aneurysm
AASLD	American Association for the Study of Liver Diseases
ACG	American College of Gastroenterology
ADPKD	Autosomal dominant polycystic kidney disease
AFB	Acid-fast bacilli
AFP	Alpha-fetoprotein
AGA	American Gastroenterological Association
AIDS	Acquired immunodeficiency syndrome
AIH	Autoimmune hepatitis
ALP	Alkaline phosphatase
ALT	Alanine aminotransferase
AMA	Anti-mitochondria antibody
ANA	Anti-nuclear antibodies
ANC	Acute necrotic collection
APC	Adenomatous polyposis coli
APC	Argon plasma coagulation
APFC	Acute peripancreatic fluid collection
ASCA	Anti-*Saccharomyces cerevisiae* antibody
ASGE	American Society for Gastrointestinal Endoscopy
ASMA	Anti-smooth muscle antibody
AST	Aspartate aminotransferase
AXR	Abdominal X-ray
BCG	Bacillus Calmette-Guerin
BCLC	Barcelona Clinic Liver Cancer
BE	Base excess
BP	Blood pressure
CA	Carbohydrate antigen/Cancer antigen
CBC	Complete blood count
CBD	Common bile duct

CD	Crohn's disease
CDAD	*Clostridium difficile*-associated colitis
CE	Capsule endoscopy
CEA	Carcinoembryonic antigen
CIPO	Chronic intestinal pseudo-obstruction
CLT	Cadaveric liver transplantation
CMV	*Cytomegalovirus*
CRC	Colorectal carcinoma
CRP	C-reactive protein
CT	Computed tomography
CTE	Computed tomography enteroclysis or enterography
CVVH	Continuous veno-venous haemofiltration
CXR	Chest X-ray
DCP	Des-gamma-carboxy prothrombin
DLBCL	Diffuse large B-cell lymphoma
DM	Diabetes mellitus
EASL	European Association for the Study of the Liver
ECCO	European Crohn's and Colitis Organisation
ECG	Electrocardiography
ECMO	Extracorporeal membrane oxygenation
EIM	Extra-intestinal manifestations
ELISA	Enzyme-linked immunosorbent assay
EMR	Endoscopic mucosal resection
ENKL	Extranodal NK/T-cell lymphoma
ERCP	Endoscopic retrograde cholangiopancreatography
ESD	Endoscopic submucosal dissection
ESR	Erythrocyte sedimentation rate
ESWL	Extracorporeal shock-wave lithotripsy
EUS	Endoscopic ultrasound
FAP	Familial adenomatous polyposis
Fe	Iron
FGP	Fundic gland polyps
FMT	Faecal microbiota transplantation
FNA	Fine-needle aspiration

FNAC	Fine-needle aspiration for cytology
FOB	Faecal occult blood
GAVE	Gastric antral vascular ectasia
GCS	Glasgow Coma Scale
GGT	Gamma-glutamyltransferase
GI	Gastrointestinal
GIB	Gastrointestinal bleeding
GIST	Gastrointestinal stromal tumour
GOJ	Gastro-oesophageal junction
GOO	Gastric outlet obstruction
GORD	Gastro-oesophageal reflux disease
Hb	Haemoglobin
HBV	Hepatitis B virus
HCC	Hepatocellular carcinoma
HCV	Hepatitis C virus
HER-2	Human epidermal growth factor receptor type 2
HIV	Human immunodeficiency virus
HNPCC	Hereditary non-polyposis colorectal cancer
HP	*Helicobacter pylori*
HR	Heart rate
HRM	High-resolution manometry
HS	Heart sounds
HS	Hyperinfection syndrome
HTLV-I	Human T-lymphotropic virus type I
IBD	Inflammatory bowel disease
ICU	Intensive care unit
IEE	Image-enhanced endoscopy
IgG	Immunoglobulin G
IGRA	Interferon-γ release assays
IHD	Intrahepatic duct
INR	International Normalised Ratio
IPMN	Intraductal papillary mucinous neoplasm
ITB	Intestinal tuberculosis
IV	Intravenous

K+	Potassium
LDH	Lactate dehydrogenase
LDLT	Living donor liver transplantation
LFT	Liver function test
LN	Lymph node
LOS	Lower oesophageal sphincter
MALT	Mucosa-associated lymphoid tissue
MCN	Mucinous cystic neoplasm
MCV	Mean corpuscular volume
MEN	Multiple endocrine neoplasia
ML	Mechanical lithotripsy
MPD	Main pancreatic duct
MRE	Magnetic resonance enteroclysis or enterography
MRI	Magnetic resonance imaging
MTB-PCR	*Mycobacterium tuberculosis* — polymerase chain reaction
Na+	Sodium
NAFLD	Non-alcoholic fatty liver disease
NET	Neuroendocrine tumour
NME	Necrolytic migratory erythema
NSAID	Non-steroidal anti-inflammatory drug
NSF	Nephrogenic systemic fibrosis
OA	Osteoarthritis
OC	Occlusion cholangiogram
OGD	Oesophagogastroduodenoscopy
OGIB	Obscure gastrointestinal bleeding
OGJ	Oesophagogastric junction
OTC	Over the counter
PAS	Periodic acid Schiff
PBC	Primary biliary cirrhosis
PCLD	Polycystic liver disease
PD	Pneumatic dilatation
PDAC	Pancreatic ductal adenocarcinoma
PEI	Percutaneous ethanol injection
PET-CT	Positron emission tomography with computed tomography

PG	Pyoderma gangrenosum
PHG	Hypertensive gastropathy
POEM	Peroral endoscopic myotomy
PPI	Proton pump inhibitor
PRRT	Peptide receptor radionuclide therapy
PSC	Primary sclerosing cholangitis
PST	Performance status test
PWON	Pancreatic walled-off necrosis
RA	Room air
RFA	Radiofrequency ablation
RFS	Recurrence-free survival
RFT	Renal function test
RPC	Recurrent pyogenic cholangitis
RUT	Rapid urease test
SCC	Squamous cell carcinoma
SCN	Serous cystic neoplasm
SEMS	Self-expandable metallic stent
SMA	Smooth muscle antibody
SPT	Solid pseudopapillary tumour
SSA	Somatostatin analogue
sTSH	Serum thyroid-stimulating hormone
TACE	Transarterial chemoembolisation
TB	Tuberculosis
TIBC	Total iron-binding capacity
TNF	Tumour necrosis factor
UC	Ulcerative colitis
USG	Ultrasonography
WBC	White blood cell
WHO	World Health Organization
ZN	Ziehl-Neelsen

Acknowledgements

We would like to acknowledge our mentors, brother and sisters within the gastroenterology and hepatology team, CUHK, for their care and dedication to the patients.

Professor Joseph Sung

Professor Francis Chan

Professor Henry Chan

Professor Justin Wu

Professor Vincent Wong

Professor Grace Wong

Professor Sunny Wong

Dr. Raymond Tang

Dr. Joyce Mak

Dr. Ting Ting Chan

Dr. Louis Lau

Dr. John Wong

Dr. Moe Kyaw

Dedication

To my wonderful family — where would I be without your support and love. To my little ones Olivia and Oscar — your growth is my constant source of joy and pride. To my teachers, Francis, Joseph and Justin — your vision enriched me with hope and wisdom. To my students — with you I learn more every day.

SCN

Dedication of this book goes to my gorgeous wife, Agnes, for always standing beside me through my ups and downs, for her endless, unconditional love and for being my soulmate. I would also like to dedicate this book to my wonderful family — my amazing dad and mum for their unfailing support and guidance through every phase of my life and my lovely brother for being my best mate. Last but not least, dedication goes to my mentors, fellow colleagues, students and patients for constantly inspiring me to be a better doctor.

HC

To my lovely daughter, Kaylee and loving wife, Tina, who bear witness to this writing journey coinciding with several of life's most important milestones.

RL

Case 1

History

A 53-year-old Chinese man with previous good health presented with a 6-month history of diarrhoea, weight loss, poor appetite and malaise. Colonoscopy showed a 40cm long segment of cobblestoning, with circumferential narrowing and ulceration in the descending colon highly suspicious for colorectal malignancy (Figure 1.1). A left hemicolectomy was performed. Histology showed ulcer exudates with granulation tissue. It was negative for malignancy and tuberculosis. He was well for 3 months after the operation, but now presents again with increasing diarrhoea up to 3-4 times per day, together with painful swallowing and tongue pain.

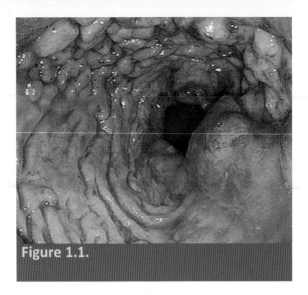

Figure 1.1.

What is your differential diagnosis?

The differential diagnosis includes Crohn's disease, malignancy, tuberculosis of the intestinal tract and Behçet's disease.

Physical examination

- Temperature 37.7°C, pulse 80 bpm, BP 120/75mmHg, SaO$_2$ 99% on RA.
- Mild pallor.
- Examination of the hands reveals no clubbing and normal-appearing palmar creases.
- On examination of the head and neck, there is a left tongue base mass with ulceration and right supraclavicular lymph nodes which are firm in consistency and around 1cm in size.
- Cardiovascular: HS dual, no murmur.
- His chest is clear on auscultation.
- Abdominal examination reveals a midline laparotomy scar. The abdomen is soft, non-tender, with no definite abdominal mass palpable.
- No signs of oedema.

Does this narrow your differential diagnosis?

Recurrence of colorectal malignancy is less likely in this context as metastatic lymph nodes will more commonly cause enlargement of the left supraclavicular lymph node, i.e. Virchow's node (Troisier's sign). However, the lymph nodes and tongue base lesion are also atypical for Crohn's disease. Initial testing for tuberculosis is also negative and there are no other features suggestive of Behçet's disease.

Investigations

- CBC:
    - WBC 11.9 x 10^9/L;
    - haemoglobin 10.9g/dL (microcytic, hypochromic picture);
    - platelets 348 x 10^9/L.
- ESR 67mm/hr.
- CRP 64.5mg/L.

What other blood tests would you order?

- Liver and renal function tests.
- Bone profile.
- Iron profile. This shows an iron deficiency picture.

What do these laboratory data suggest?

These laboratory findings suggest active inflammation with suspected iron deficiency anaemia.

What imaging test would you order?

With the presence of a tongue base mass with ulceration, it is important to arrange for imaging to assess any deep tissue involvement. For better soft tissue resolution, magnetic resonance imaging (MRI) of the neck is arranged (Figure 1.2).

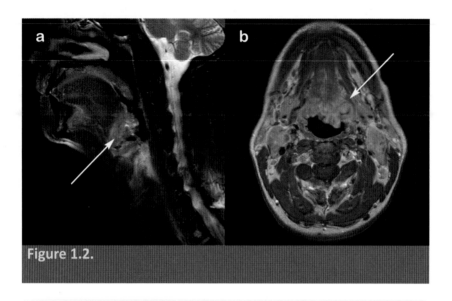

Figure 1.2.

Please describe what you see

An MRI of the neck shows a left tongue base mass measuring 4cm x 2.7cm x 3.4cm, with unusual findings of ulceration and an exophytic frond-like appearance. There is also inferior extension involving the lower left lateral oropharyngeal wall and valleculae. Bilateral enlarged nodes in the upper, mid and lower internal jugular chains are also noted.

How would you proceed?

An excisional biopsy of the right neck lymph node should be arranged.

Histology shows multiple patches of necrosis surrounded by lymphohistiocytic infiltrate, superficially resembling necrotising granulomatous inflammation.

What is your differential diagnosis for necrotising lymphadenitis?

Infection
- Disseminated mycobacterium infection.
- Cat scratch disease.
- *Yersinia* infection.

Autoimmune
- Crohn's disease.
- Vasculitis, i.e. eosinophilic granulomatosis with polyangiitis, granulomatosis with polyangiitis.
- Sarcoidosis.
- Kikuchi-Fujimoto disease.

Malignancy
- Lymphoma.

In view of the atypical history, physical examination and histopathological features, further immunostaining and investigations are done.

Immunostain for CD56 (natural killer NK cell marker) shows moderate numbers of small- to medium-sized lymphoid cells in the interfollicular zone, which are easily overlooked in light microscopy. These atypical lymphoid cells co-express for CD3 and CD2 but not CD5 and CD7, and are also highlighted with *in situ* hybridisation for Epstein-Barr virus (EBV) encoded RNAs.

Review of the original colonic resection also demonstrates lymphomatous infiltrates (Figure 1.3).

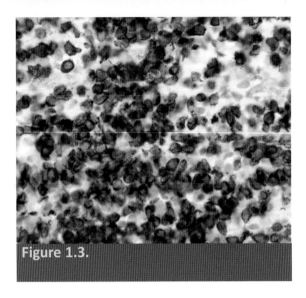

Figure 1.3.

What is the diagnosis, and how would you proceed?

Overall, the features are mostly consistent with NK/T-cell lymphoma.

The next step would be for timely referral to an oncologist for further work-up and management.

Clinical pearls

- Although rare, extranodal NK/T-cell lymphomas are more common in East Asia and South America. It is an uncommon differential diagnosis for inflammatory bowel disease especially in the older patient. A high index of clinical suspicion is required.
- Staging of a lymphoma is usually done with positron emission tomography with computed tomography (PET-CT)(Figure 1.4).

PET-CT shows right cervical lymph node involvement, lymphoma infiltrates at the base of the tongue, a hypermetabolic sigmoid tumour, nodal metastases in the left para-aortic region and generalised marrow hypermetabolism. A subsequent bone marrow exam is negative for lymphomatous infiltration.

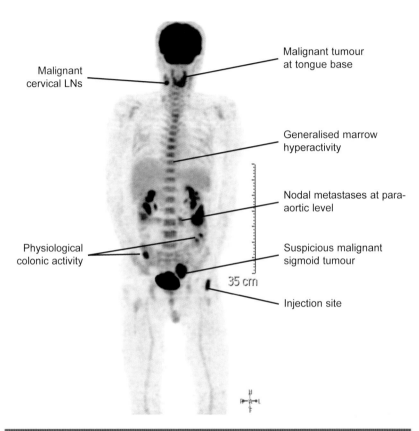

Malignant cervical LNs

Malignant tumour at tongue base

Generalised marrow hyperactivity

Nodal metastases at para-aortic level

Physiological colonic activity

Suspicious malignant sigmoid tumour

35 cm

Injection site

Figure 1.4.

Impress your attending

What virus is implicated as a possible cause for NK/T-cell lymphoma?
Epstein-Barr virus infection [1].

What is the prevalence of extranodal NK/T-cell lymphomas in East Asia?

Extranodal NK/T-cell lymphoma (ENKL) has a greater prevalence in East Asia and South America [2] compared with other parts of the world, with an occurrence rate in Asia of 3.3-8%. The majority of tumours arise from the nasal and paranasal areas. Gut involvement is rare.

What is the prognosis of non-nasal NK/T-cell lymphoma?

Prognosis is generally poor despite treatment with chemotherapy, with clinical remission in less than 15% of patients.

What do you know about the SMILE regimen?

It is a regimen using dexamethasone, methotrexate, ifosfamide, L-asparaginase and etoposide for the treatment of NK/T-cell lymphoma. It can be used in combination with radiotherapy in selected patients [3].

References

1. Kwong YL, Chan AC, Liang R, *et al.* CD56+ NK lymphomas: clinicopathological features and prognosis. *Br J Haematol* 1997; 97: 821-9.
2. Chan JK, Quintanilla-Martilla L, Ferry JA, *et al.* Extranodal NK/T-cell lymphoma, nasal type. In: Swerdlow SH, Campo E, Harris NL, *et al,* Eds. *WHO classification of tumours of haematopoietic and lymphoid tissues.* Lyon, France: IARC Press; 2008: 285-8.
3. Kwong YL, Kim WS, Lim ST, *et al.* SMILE for natural killer/T-cell lymphoma: analysis of safety and efficacy from the Asia Lymphoma Study Group. *Blood* 2012; 120(15): 2973-80.

Case 2

A 27-year-old Chinese gentleman with previous good health presents to a private physician with a 6-month history of cramping abdominal discomfort, diarrhoea up to 5-6 times per day and rectal bleeding. This is associated with weight loss of around 3-4kg over the past 6 months. He is a non-smoker and non-drinker. There is no family history of colorectal cancer or inflammatory bowel disease. He has no significant travel history. There are no recent significant life stressors.

Physical examination

- Afebrile, pulse 74 bpm, BP 110/60mmHg, SaO_2 98% on RA.
- Appears well.
- Examination of the hands reveals no clubbing and normal-appearing palmar creases.
- Head and neck examination is unremarkable.
- Cardiovascular: HS dual, no murmur.
- His chest is clear on auscultation.
- Abdominal examination reveals a soft abdomen, with no focal tenderness and no organomegaly.
- No signs of oedema.

Investigations

- CBC:
  - WBC 8.3 x 10^9/L;
  - haemoglobin 12.3g/dL (microcytic hypochromic picture);
  - platelets 255 x 10^9/L.
- ESR 31mm/hr.
- CRP 32mg/L.

What is your differential diagnosis?

The differential diagnosis includes inflammatory bowel disease and infectious colitis.

What other blood tests would you order?

- Liver and renal function tests
- Bone profile.

All are within normal limits.

What do these laboratory data suggest?

The blood work is highly suggestive of an active inflammatory process.

What other tests would you order?

An oesophagogastroduodenoscopy (OGD) and a colonoscopy are arranged.

Colonoscopic findings show multiple irregular ulcers at the transverse colon, descending colon, sigmoid colon and upper rectum. There is also terminal ileum ulceration.

Multiple biopsies are taken which show granulomatous inflammation but no acid-fast bacilli on Ziehl-Neelsen stain. No *Mycobacterium tuberculosis* polymerase chain reaction (MTB-PCR) had been performed by the previous referring hospital.

Oesophagogastroduodenoscopy shows gastritis only.

What imaging test would you order?

A CT of the abdomen and pelvis with contrast (Figure 2.1).

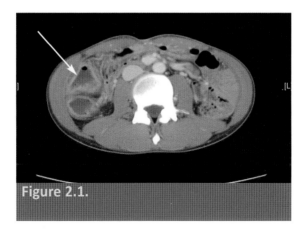

Figure 2.1.

Please describe what you see

A CT of the abdomen and pelvis with contrast shows circumferential wall thickening and oedema at the hepatic flexure, ascending colon, caecum and terminal ileum (arrow). The hepatic flexure and ascending colon are most severely affected. There is associated hypervascular mesentery and reactive mesenteric lymph nodes. These features are suggestive of active inflammatory change.

There is no evidence of abscess or fistula formation.

What is your diagnosis, and how would you proceed?

The clinical picture is compatible with ileocolonic Crohn's disease.

He is started on prednisolone and azathioprine, and is planned for early clinic follow-up for review of progress.

The patient has good compliance to medications, but there is no improvement in his symptoms for 1 month. He then develops fever, increasing cough and sputum, with worsening abdominal pain and diarrhoea for 3 weeks prior to hospital admission. There is subjective weight loss and poor appetite. Symptoms of night sweats, fever and haemoptysis are negative.

Physical examination shows a fever of 38°C. Chest examination reveals right upper zone inspiratory crepitations.

What would you do next?

The new onset of chest symptoms and fever after the use of immunosuppressives warrant thorough investigation and treatment. There is also a lack of response to treatment with worsening abdominal symptoms.

Admission and a chest X-ray are arranged (Figure 2.2).

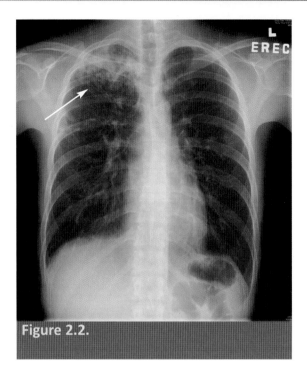

Figure 2.2.

Please describe what you see

A chest X-ray (Figure 2.2) shows right upper lobe infiltrates. Repeat bloods also show an erythrocyte sedimentation rate of up to 70mm/hr.

What is your differential diagnosis?

Secondary chest infection due to immunosuppression and disseminated tuberculosis.

How would you manage this patient?

- Stop the immunosuppressants.
- Start empirical antibiotics.
- Save sputum for culture, acid-fast bacilli staining and TB culture.

- Arrange for bronchoscopy and bronchoscopic alveolar lavage.
- Repeat colonoscopy.

Bronchoscopy shows whitish lesions over the right basal segment. Lavage is sent for Gram stain and culture, acid-fast bacilli and tuberculosis culture (AFB and TB culture), MTB-PCR, fungal cultures and cytology.

Repeat colonoscopy shows similar findings as before. Multiple biopsies are taken again. Histology shows necrotising granulomas. Specimens are also sent for Gram stain and culture, AFB and TB culture, and MTB-PCR.

AFB stains were negative all along. Subsequently, *Mycobacterium tuberculosis* DNA is positive from both colonic and lung specimens, and tuberculosis cultures are also positive after 8 weeks.

Anti-tuberculosis treatment is initiated. The patient is seen in clinic around 1 month later. Gastrointestinal symptoms are improving with less abdominal pain and diarrhoea, and no more per rectal bleeding. His body weight increases to 47kg from 40kg and his inflammatory markers are on a downward trend.

Clinical pearls

- The differentiation of Crohn's disease and tuberculosis of the intestinal tract, especially in endemic regions and in the early phase, is challenging.
- Close monitoring and follow-up with a high index of suspicion is often required to arrive at the definitive diagnosis.

Impress your attending

How common is tuberculosis of the intestinal tract?
Tuberculosis of the gut is uncommon. In 2011, there were a total of 4794 new cases of tuberculosis in Hong Kong, of which 91 had

involvement of either the peritoneum, intestines, mesentery or appendix, accounting for around 1.9% of cases [1].

What are the risk factors for tuberculosis of the intestinal tract?
- Advanced age.
- Low socioeconomic status.
- HIV [2].
- Alcoholic liver disease.

What is the presentation of intestinal tuberculosis?
It can mainly be divided into ulcerative and hyperplastic types. The ulcerative type usually has mucosal ulceration, bleeding, a risk of perforation, fistulation and stricture formation. The hyperplastic type presents with inflammatory masses and obstruction [3].

What is the duration of anti-tuberculosis treatment if the gut is affected?
An initial phase of four drugs is recommended in the first 2 months: isoniazid, rifampicin, pyrazinamide and either ethambutol or streptomycin. In the continuation phase, usually only two drugs are given: isoniazid and rifampicin — usually for 4-7 months, for a total treatment duration of 6-9 months.

Do you know of any new drugs for the treatment of tuberculosis [4]?
- Delamanid. It acts by blocking the synthesis of mycolic acids in *Mycobacterium tuberculosis* leading to destabilisation of its cell wall.
- Bedaquiline. It acts by inhibiting mycobacterial ATP synthetase and depletes cellular energy stores.

References

1. Tuberculosis and Chest Service of the Department of Health. Annual report, 2011. Hong Kong Special Administrative Region.
2. Corbett EL, Watt CJ, Walker N, *et al*. The growing burden of tuberculosis: global trends and interactions with the HIV epidemic. *Arch Intern Med* 2003; 163: 1009-21.

3.   Aston NO. Abdominal tuberculosis. *World J Surg* 1997; 21: 492-9.

4.   Zumla A, Chakaya J, Centis R, *et al*. Tuberculosis treatment and management - an update on treatment regimens, trials, new drugs, and adjunct therapies. *Lancet Respir Med* 2015; 3(3): 220-34.

Case 3

History

A 51-year-old gentleman initially presented with loose bowel motions and abdominal pain in 2008. He had a past history of peptic ulcer disease treated with a partial gastrectomy. Private colonoscopy showed ileocecal colitis. Colonic biopsy showed acid-fast bacilli on staining, but culture for tuberculosis was negative. Anti-tuberculosis treatment was commenced for a duration of 10 months. Upon follow-up, repeat colonoscopy still showed ileocecal valve ulceration. Repeat biopsy was negative for acid-fast bacilli and tuberculosis DNA polymerase chain reaction (TB-PCR).

He has now been referred to a tertiary hospital in view of worsening symptoms of abdominal cramps and bowel opening up to three times per day. He also complains of loss of appetite and weight loss of around 1kg in the past month. He has no symptoms of gastrointestinal bleeding, and also no mucus per rectum. He denies any oral or genital ulcers, joint pain or eye symptoms.

What is your differential diagnosis?

The differential diagnosis includes intestinal tuberculosis (ITB), Crohn's disease (CD) and Behçet's disease.

Physical examination

- Afebrile, pulse 90 bpm, BP 134/72mmHg, SaO_2 98% on RA.
- Hydration is satisfactory.
- Examination of the hands reveals no clubbing and normal-appearing palmar creases.
- On examination of the head and neck, the oral cavity is normal with no ulceration.
- Cardiovascular: HS dual, no murmur.
- His chest is clear on auscultation.
- Abdominal examination reveals a soft abdomen, with tenderness over the right lower quadrant and no definite mass.
- No signs of oedema.

Does this narrow your differential diagnosis? What diagnosis does the physical examination suggest?

Yes. The lack of mucosal ulceration on physical examination and no history of symptoms suggestive of uveitis or skin pathergy are less suggestive of Behçet's disease.

Investigations

- CBC:
  - WBC 10 x 10^9/L;
  - haemoglobin 10.4g/dL;
  - platelets 369 x 10^9/L.
- ESR 46mm/hr.
- CRP 51mg/L.
- Liver and renal function tests are grossly normal.

What other blood tests would you order?

- Iron profile: Fe 4μmol/L, TIBC 26μmol/L, Fe 14%.

What do these laboratory data suggest?

Active inflammation with iron deficiency anaemia; the origin may be from the gastrointestinal tract.

How would you proceed?

In view of worsening symptoms and poor response to previous treatment, a repeat colonoscopy should be arranged (Figure 3.1).

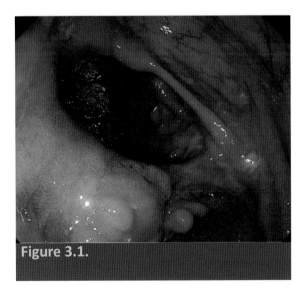

Figure 3.1.

Please describe what you see
Colonoscopy shows a distorted ileocecal valve with an overlying ulcer and inflammation. An irregular ulcer in the terminal ileum is also noted.

What imaging test would you order?

Computed tomography enteroclysis (CTE) for small bowel work-up (Figure 3.2).

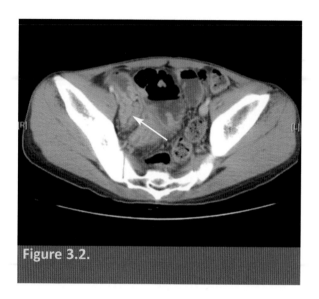

Figure 3.2.

Please describe what you see
Contrast CT shows asymmetrical wall thickening at the distal and terminal ileum associated with multiple ulcers, a mucosal polypoid appearance and contour deformity. Luminal narrowing is also noted at the abnormal segment suggestive of an inflammatory stricture.

What is the diagnosis, and how would you proceed?

With small bowel, terminal ileum and ileocecal ulceration, there is a possibility of Crohn's disease. However, biopsies show a benign ulcer only without other characteristic features. Repeated acid-fast bacilli (AFB) and TB culture are negative.

Empirical Crohn's disease treatment with high-dose intravenous steroids is started. However, his symptoms worsen and a repeat colonoscopy is performed. Similar ulcers are seen and histology reveals a small non-caseating granuloma with no other features of inflammatory bowel disease. Periodic acid Schiff (PAS), Ziehl-Neelsen (ZN), TB-PCR and immunostains for *Cytomegalovirus* (CMV) are all negative. Prednisolone is stopped and empirical TB treatment is given. He does not respond with persistent right lower quadrant, abdominal pain, an increasing ESR, decreasing albumin to 27g/L, and worsening anaemia to 6.4g/dL.

What is the next step?

The surgical team is consulted and a right hemicolectomy for diagnostic and therapeutic purposes is arranged. Intra-operatively, a grossly oedematous and erythematous terminal ileum is noted. A surgical specimen shows benign ulcerations and deep fissures, in keeping with Crohn's disease. TB-PCR and culture are negative.

He is started on prednisolone and azathioprine.

Upon follow-up he has no further symptoms, with improving body weight and biochemical parameters. His latest Hb is 12.9g/dL and his inflammatory markers are normal.

Clinical pearls

- The differentiation between Crohn's disease and intestinal tuberculosis (ITB) can be difficult as illustrated in the above case.
- On rare occasions, surgical resection is needed to make the definitive diagnosis and treatment.

Impress your attending

What is the definition of a granuloma?
It is defined as an organised collection of epithelioid macrophages.

How would you distinguish between Crohn's disease and ITB (Table 3.1)?

Table 3.1. Distinguishing between Crohn's disease and ITB.

	Crohn's disease	ITB
Duration of symptoms	May be longer (12 months)	May be shorter (6 months)
Perianal disease	More suggestive	Less suggestive
Chest symptoms	Less suggestive	More suggestive
ELISA against ASCA	More likely positive	More likely negative
TB culture	Negative	Positive
MTB-PCR	Negative	Positive
QuantiFERON-TB	More likely negative	More likely positive
Endoscopy	More suggestive of Crohn's: aphthoid or longitudinal deep fissuring ulcers, fistulation, cobblestone appearance, skip lesions	More suggestive of ITB: transverse placed ulcers, nodularity, hypertrophic lesions resembling masses
Biopsy	Non-caseating granulomas AFB negative	Caseating granulomas AFB positive

MTB-PCR: *Mycobacterium tuberculosis* — polymerase chain reaction.
ELISA: enzyme-linked immunosorbent assay.
ASCA: anti-*Saccharomyces cerevisiae* antibody.

Below is a proposed algorithm for the assessment and treatment for these patients (Figure 3.3) [1].

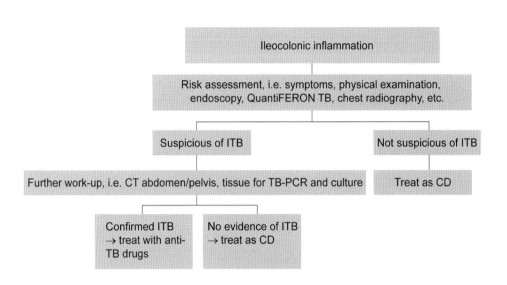

ITB: intestinal tuberculosis.
CD: Crohn's disease.
CT: computed tomography.
PCR: polymerase chain reaction.

Figure 3.3. An algorithm for the assessment and treatment of patients with ileocolonic inflammation.

References

1. Almadi MA, Ghosh S, Abdulrahman M. Differentiating intestinal tuberculosis from Crohn's disease: a diagnostic challenge. *Am J Gastroenterol* 2009; 104(4): 1003-12.

Case 4

A 32-year-old gentleman presented with bloody diarrhoea 9 months ago. Colonoscopy revealed pancolitis and he was treated with corticosteroids. Steroid dosage was gradually tailed down and he was maintained on mesalazine treatment. He was a smoker and quitted smoking 6 months after his initial presentation due to the birth of his daughter. He presents again with bloody diarrhoea up to 10 times per day. He has a fever and mild abdominal pain.

Physical examination

- Temperature 38.3°C, fever, pulse 130 bpm, BP 100/80mmHg, SaO_2 99% on RA.
- Tired-looking, hydration on the dry side.
- Examination of the hands reveals no clubbing and normal-appearing palmar creases.
- Head and neck examination is unremarkable.
- Cardiovascular: HS dual, no murmur.
- His chest is clear on auscultation.
- Abdominal examination reveals a soft abdomen, with no peritoneal signs.
- No signs of oedema.

Investigations

- CBC for leukocytosis and thrombocythemia.
- Liver and renal function tests for electrolyte disturbance and renal impairment.
- Inflammatory markers: ESR, CRP.
- Blood for culture to rule out septicaemia in view of high fever.

Blood tests reveal thrombocytosis and raised inflammatory markers.

What is your differential diagnosis?

The differential diagnosis includes a flare up of ulcerative colitis and infectious colitis.

What other tests would you order?

- Stool for bacterial culture.
- Stool for norovirus.
- Stool for *Clostridium difficile* toxin A and B.

- A sigmoidoscopy may be considered (AVOID full colonoscopy as there is a high risk of perforation).
- Abdominal X-ray to rule out toxic megacolon.

How would you assess the severity of the flare?

The severity of an acute ulcerative colitis flare can be assessed by the Truelove and Witts' criteria, as outlined below in Table 4.1 [1].

Table 4.1. The Truelove and Witts' criteria.			
	Mild	**Moderate**	**Severe**
Bowel movements/day	<4	4-6	>6
Temperature	Normal	Slightly elevated	Markedly elevated
Heart rate	<70	70-90	>90
Haemoglobin	>11	10.5-11	<10.5
Erythrocyte sedimentation rate	<30	-	>30

How would you manage his flare?

Start intravenous hydrocortisone. In acute severe ulcerative colitis, the first-line therapy is corticosteroids and the overall response rate to steroids is 67% [2]. Steroid treatment should not be deferred while waiting for stool microbiological results.

How would you proceed?

The patient should be reviewed for response to steroids after 72 hours. In patients not responding after 3 days of corticosteroids (defined as >8 stools per day or 3-8 stools per day plus a CRP >45mg/L), the colectomy rate rises to 85% [3].

He has persistent fever and an increase in bowel frequency despite the use of IV hydrocortisone.

Stool investigation reveals positive *Clostridium difficile* toxin.

What is the first-line management?

In non-fulminant *Clostridium difficile* infection, oral vancomycin or oral fidaxomicin is the treatment of choice. In fulminant cases, oral vancomycin with intravenous metronidazole or consideration of surgery should be considered [4].

Despite treatment with metronidazole and vancomycin, the diarrhoea and fever persist.

What other medical rescue therapies are available for a steroid-refractory ulcerative colitis flare?

- Both infliximab and IV cyclosporine may be used as medical rescue therapies for steroid-refractory acute ulcerative colitis.
- Randomised controlled trials show that both rescue therapies are equally efficacious [5].

The patient does not respond to medical rescue therapy.

How would you proceed?

The surgical team should be consulted to consider a colectomy. Surgery should be considered if the patient is not responding to first-line corticosteroid and second-line therapy, and should not be delayed for more than 5 days in patients with an inadequate response, as delayed colectomy is associated with increased in-hospital mortality [6].

A laparoscopic total colectomy is performed (Figure 4.1). He is doing well now.

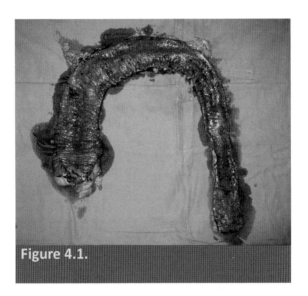

Figure 4.1.

Please describe what you see
The surgical specimen in Figure 4.1 shows severe inflammatory changes involving the entire resected colon.

Clinical pearls

- Steroids are the first-line therapy for acute severe ulcerative colitis.
- Infection has to be excluded in patients with an ulcerative colitis flare.
- *Clostridium difficile* infection is not uncommon in patients with inflammatory bowel disease and the incidence is increasing [7].

Impress your attending

What precautions are necessary to prevent the spread of the Clostridium difficile infection?
- Contact precautions.
- Wash hands under running water after contact with the patient.
- *Clostridium difficile* spores cannot be removed by alcohol-based swab, and hand washing under running water is essential [4].

References

1. Truelove SC, Witts L. Cortisone in ulcerative colitis: final report on a therapeutic trial. *BMJ* 1955; 2: 1041-8.
2. Turner D, Walsh CM, Steinhart AH, Griffiths AM. Response to corticosteroid in severe ulcerative colitis: a systemic review of the literature and a meta-regression. *Clin Gastroenterol Hepatol* 2007; 5: 103-10.
3. Travis SP, Farrant JM, Ricketts C, *et al*. Predicting outcome in severe ulcerative colitis. *Gut* 1996; 38: 905-10.
4. https://academic.oup.com/cid/article/66/7/e1/4855916.
5. Dean KE, Hikaka J, Huakau JT, Walmsley RS. Infliximab or cyclosporine for acute severe ulcerative colitis: a retrospective analysis. *J Gastroenterol Hepatol* 2012; 27: 487-92.
6. Kaplan G, McCarthy EP, Ayanian JZ, *et al*. Impact of hospital volume on postoperative morbidity and mortality following a colectomy for ulcerative colitis. *Gastroenterol* 2008; 134: 680-7.
7. Ananthakrishnan AN, Issa M, Binion DG. *Clostridium difficile* and inflammatory bowel disease. *Med Clin North Am* 2010; 94: 135-53.

Case 5

History

A 27-year-old gentleman with ileocolonic Crohn's disease and perianal involvement has previously been well controlled with azathioprine. He had an episode of disease flare and was started on infliximab for treatment of his active lumimal disease. His tuberculin skin test was negative and his chest X-ray was normal prior to starting an anti-TNF agent. Two weeks after starting infliximab, he develops a fever up to 38.5°C.

Physical examination

- Fever 38.9°C, haemodynamically stable, SaO_2 98-100% on RA.
- Hydration is satisfactory.
- Examination of the hands reveals no clubbing and normal-appearing palmar creases.
- Head and neck examination is unremarkable.
- Cardiovascular: HS dual, no murmur.
- Chest examination reveals crepitations and decreased air entry in the left upper zone.
- Abdominal examination reveals a soft, non-tender abdomen.
- Perianal examination reveals no active perianal disease or signs of infection.
- No signs of oedema.

Investigations

- CBC is normal.
- Liver function tests are normal (for preparation of future anti-TB treatment).
- ESR >120mm/hr.
- CRP 200mg/L.

What are the possible causes of his fever given his history of Crohn's?

- Infective causes (with the use of immunosuppressive therapy, there is a high risk of infection. Infective causes must be considered in patients on immunosuppressive therapy. In Asia, with the high prevalence of tuberculosis [TB], reactivation of latent TB must be ruled out):
  - intra-abdominal collections;
  - perianal abscess;
  - opportunistic infections due to underlying immunosuppression;
  - reactivation of TB or active TB.
- Fever due to underlying active Crohn's disease.

What further investigations would you perform?

- Chest imaging (chest X-ray or CT thorax) to confirm the presence of consolidation (Figure 5.1).
- Sputum for routine culture.
- Sputum for Ziehl-Neelsen (ZN) stain and TB culture.

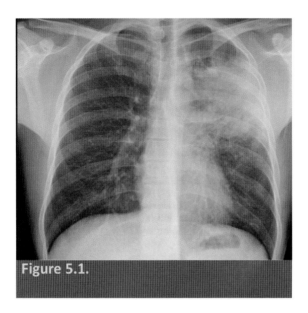

Figure 5.1.

Please describe what you see
There are consolidative changes with infiltrates and an air bronchogram in the left upper lobe.

Later on, the ZN stain shows acid-fast bacilli. How would this affect your management?

The presence of acid-fast bacilli is consistent with the diagnosis of open TB. It is highly contagious and airborne isolation precautions is warranted.

Tuberculosis is a slow-growing organism and usually takes more than a month to grow. Empirical anti-TB treatment should be commenced and subsequently adjusted according to the sensitivity when the culture result is available.

As TB is an acquired immunodeficiency syndrome (AIDS) defining illness, human immunodeficiency virus (HIV) status should also be checked.

Clinical pearls

- Latent TB must be screened before the initiation of immunosuppressive therapy.
- The use of immunosuppressive therapy may cause a false-negative result of the tuberculin skin test.

Impress your attending

How would you screen for TB?

The European Crohn's and Colitis Organisation (ECCO) guidelines on the screening of opportunistic infection in IBD suggest screening of latent TB based on epidemiological risk factors, physical examination, chest X-ray, and an interferon-gamma release assay and/or a tuberculin skin test [1].

What are the possible causes of a false-negative Mantoux test?

- A tuberculin skin test may be negative in patients on corticosteroids for >1 month, or thiopurines or methotrexate for >3 months [1].
- It may also occur during active IBD without immunosuppression [1].
- HIV infection may also be a cause.

What can cause a false-positive Mantoux test result?

- A previous Bacillus Calmette-Guerin (BCG) vaccination may cause a false-positive result [1].

What is the performance of interferon-γ release assays in the diagnosis of latent TB (Table 5.1 [2])?

- Interferon-γ release assays (IGRA) target two specific proteins of *M. tuberculosis* (ESAT-6 and CFP-10).

- These are not affected by BCG-vaccination or environmental mycobacterial exposure.

Table 5.1. Comparison of tests used for latent TB.

	IGRA	Tuberculin skin test
Sensitivity (%)	~80-90	~80
Specificity (%):		
• Non-BCG-vaccinated	>95	>95
• BCG-vaccinated	>95	~60

What would be your approach if the patient has latent tuberculosis?
- Isoniazid monotherapy can be given to the patient.
- It offers 90% protection provided by the completion of a 9-month course.

What are the potential side effects from the therapy?
- Hepatotoxicity.
- Peripheral neuropathy (can be prevented with the co-administration of pyridoxine) [3].

References

1. Rahier JF, Ben-Horin S, Chowers Y, *et al.* European evidence-based Consensus on the prevention, diagnosis and management of opportunistic infections in inflammatory bowel disease. *J Crohn's Colitis* 2009; 3: 47-91.
2. Blumberg HM, Kempker RR. Interferon-γ release assays for the evaluation of tuberculosis infection. *JAMA* 2014; 312(14): 1460-1.
3. Horsburgh CR Jr, Rubin EJ. Latent tuberculosis infection in the United States. *N Engl J Med* 2011; 364(15): 1441-8.

Case 6

History

A 45-year-old lady presents with recurrent abdominal pain which she has experienced for a few years. She also complains of recurrent oral ulceration and persistent vaginal discharge and ulceration. She has no fever and denies any diarrhoea or weight loss. Colonoscopy shows a large oval-shaped ulcer in the ileum; otherwise no other colonic mucosal lesions are noted.

Physical examination

- Afebrile, pulse 72 bpm, BP 125/80mmHg, SaO_2 97% on RA.
- Her general appearance is unremarkable.
- Examination of the hands reveals no clubbing and normal-appearing palmar creases.
- Head and neck examination is unremarkable and no cervical lymph nodes are palpable. There are multiple aphthous ulcers in the oral cavity, but no oral thrush.
- Cardiovascular: HS dual, no murmur.
- Her chest is clear on auscultation.
- Abdominal examination is unremarkable.
- No signs of oedema.

On gynaecological examination, multiple vaginal ulcers are noted on physical examination but no definite fistula openings are noted.

What is your differential diagnosis?

The differential diagnosis includes Behçet's disease, Crohn's disease and infective causes including intestinal tuberculosis and *Cytomegalovirus* (CMV) colitis.

What blood test(s) would you order?

- CBC.
- Liver function tests.
- CRP.
- ESR.

All blood tests are unremarkable.

What further investigations would you order?

A chest X-ray (Figure 6.1) and an MRI of the pelvis. A small-bowel follow-through series can also be useful (Figures 6.2-6.4). CT enterography/MR enterography are other modalities used for small bowel work-up.

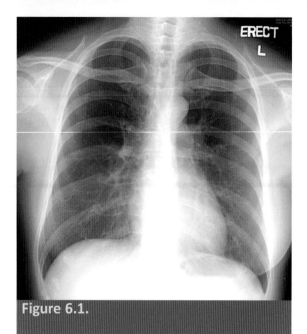

Figure 6.1.

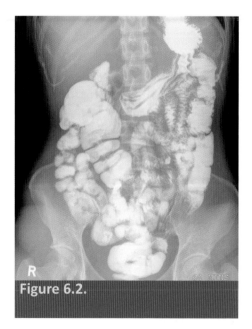

Figure 6.2.

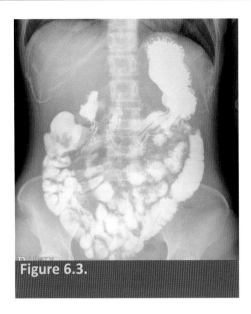

Figure 6.3.

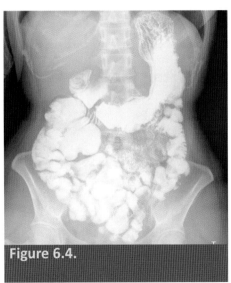

Figure 6.4.

Please describe what you see

The chest X-ray in Figure 6.1 shows a clear lung field. The small-bowel follow-through series (Figures 6.2-6.4) does not reveal any fistulae or strictures. The MRI of the pelvis (not seen here) does not reveal any fistulae.

Does this narrow your differential diagnosis?

This is more likely to be Behçet's disease.

In colonoscopy, what are the features suggestive of Behçet's disease?

The ulcers in intestinal Behçet's disease are usually oval in shape and tend to be larger and deeper [1]. The ulcers usually have discrete borders, and are located in the ileocecal area [1]. Stricture formation and fistulae are more frequently observed in cases of Crohn's disease [2].

On histological examination, what is the important feature that differentiates Crohn's from Behçet's disease?

The presence of non-caseating granuloma is highly suggestive of Crohn's disease, whereas it is an uncommon feature in intestinal Behçet's disease [2].

What is a pathergy test and how would you perform it?

It is performed by pricking the forearm with a small, sterile needle. Occurrence of a pustule at the site of needle insertion, 1-2 days after the test, constitutes a positive test. It is useful in diagnosing Behçet's disease and has a specificity of ~90% [3]. However, the rate of positive pathergy tests has been reported to be lower than 40% [3].

What other skin manifestations may be seen in Behçet's disease [4]?

- Folliculitis.
- Erythema nodosum.
- Vasculitic rash.
- Acne in post-adolescents not on corticosteroids.

What are the diagnostic criteria for Behçet's disease?

According to the International Study Group guidelines, for a patient to be diagnosed with Behçet's disease, the patient must have the 'hallmark' symptoms oulined in Table 6.1 below [4].

Table 6.1. Revised international criteria for Behçet's disease.	
Sign/symptom	**Score**
Oral aphthosis	2
Genital aphthosis	2
Ocular manifestations	2
Skin manifestations	1
Vascular manifestations	1
Central nervous system involvement	1
Positive pathergy test	1

Point score system (sensitivity 94.8% and specificity 90.5%; if the pathergy test is included, the sensitivity and specificity increases to 98.5% and 91.6%, respectively). A score of ≥4 indicates Behçet's disease.
Pathergy testing is optional and the primary scoring system does not include pathergy testing. However, where pathergy testing is conducted, 1 extra point may be assigned for a positive result.

What are the treatment options for Behçet's disease?

* Topical steroids for mouth ulcers.
* Thalidomide.
* Azathioprine.
* Colchicine or interferon for mucocutanoues manifestations.
* Systemic steroids for uveitis.

The patient is started with colchicine and she has prompt improvement of GI symptoms and remains well.

Clinical pearls

- Behçet's disease was originally described in 1937 and is characterised by oral and genital ulceration, and ocular inflammation [5].

Impress your attending

How frequent are GI symptoms in patients with Behçet's disease?
Over 40% of patients may have GI symptoms [6]. The most frequent area of involvement in GI Behçet's disease is the ileocecal region with extension into the ascending colon, with only 15% having diffuse involvement of the colon [7]. Patients typically have a few (<5) ulcers oval in shape, deep, with discrete borders, and located in the ileocecal area [1].

References

1. Lee SK, Kim BK, Kim TI, *et al.* Differential diagnosis of intestinal Behçet's disease and Crohn's disease by colonoscopic findings. *Endoscopy* 2009; 41: 9-16.
2. Lakhanpal S, Tani K, Lie JT, *et al.* Pathologic features of Behçet's syndrome: a review of Japanese autopsy registry data. *Hum Pathol* 1985; 16: 790-5.
3. Chang HK, Cheon KS. The clinical significance of a pathergy reaction in patients with Behçet's disease. *J Korean Med Sci* 2002; 17: 371-4.
4. International Team for the Revision of the International Criteria for Behçet's Disease (ITR-ICBD). The International Criteria for Behçet's Disease (ICBD): a collaborative study of 27 countries on the sensitivity and specificity of the new criteria. *J Eur Acad Dermatol Venereol* 2014; 28(3): 338-47.
5. Behçet H. Uber rezidivierende, aphthose, durch ein virus verursachte Geschwure am Mund, am Auge und an den Genitalien. *Dermatol Wochenschr* 1937; 105: 1152-7.
6. Kasahara Y, Tanaka S, Nihino M, *et al.* Intestinal involvement in Behçet's disease: review of 136 surgical cases in the Japanese literature. *Dis Colon Rectum* 1981; 24: 103-6.
7. Mizushima Y, Inaba G, Mimura Y. Diagnostic criteria for Behçet's disease in 1987, and guideline for treating Behçet's disease. *Saishin Igaku* 1988; 43: 391-3.

Case 7

History

A 54-year-old gentleman who drank half a bottle of vodka daily for over 20 years presents with severe epigastric pain and a bilateral lower limb violaceous skin rash for 1 week. This is associated with fever and confusion.

Physical examination

- Temperature 38.2°C, pulse 120 bpm, BP 120/78mmHg, SaO_2 95% on RA.
- Hydration on the dry side.
- Examination of the hands reveals no clubbing, palmar erythema and a hepatic flap.
- Head and neck examination is unremarkable.
- Cardiovascular: HS dual, no murmur.
- His chest is clear on auscultation.
- Abdominal examination reveals a central tenderness, but no guarding/rebound tenderness.
- GCS 14/15 with confused speech and disorientation; otherwise there is no focal neurological deficit detected.
- Mild lower limb oedema is noted.

Figure 7.1 is a clinical photo of his lower limb rash.

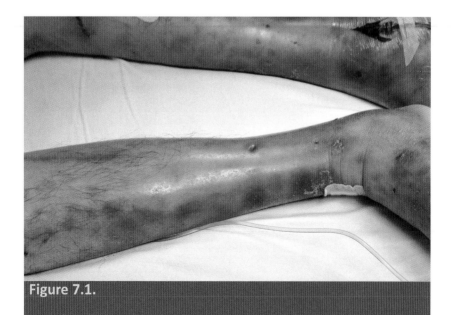

Figure 7.1.

Please describe what you see

A violaceous, slightly indurated, tender maculopapular rash has developed over his lower limbs.

Investigations

- CBC:
    - WBC 33 x 10^9/L;
    - haemoglobin 12g/dL;
    - platelets 255 x 10^9/L.
- Amylase 1058 IU/L.
- Liver and renal function tests are normal.
- International Normalised Ratio is normal.

What are the potential causes for the skin lesions?

- Septic emboli to skin (i.e. meningococcal septicaemia).
- Erythema nodosum.
- Pancreatic panniculitis.
- Drug eruption.

Given the raised amylase in this clinical context, panniculitis associated with pancreatitis is the most likely diagnosis.

How would you manage this patient?

- Supportive care with aggressive fluid resuscitation and close monitoring of vital signs.
- Early enteral nutrition [1].
- Analgesics.
- +/- Antibiotics (controversial) [2].

Despite the above measures, this patient continues to have severe abdominal pain and high fever. Subsequently he develops shock with a blood pressure of 80/60mmHg. Haemoglobin drops by 2g/dL. He is admitted to the intensive care unit for further care and close monitoring.

What further investigations would you request?

Computed tomography (CT) scans of the abdomen and pelvis with contrast should be done (Figures 7.2 and 7.3).

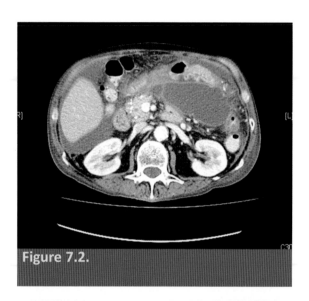

Figure 7.2.

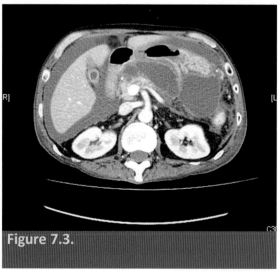

Figure 7.3.

Please describe what you see

The CT images show multiple punctuated calcifications at the head of the pancreas. Moderate-sized loculated fluid collections are seen lying anterior to the body and tail of the pancreas. There is high-density blood present in the pseudocyst and in the lesser sac. No ongoing contrast extravasation is noted.

An emergency laparotomy is done. Intra-operatively, a large volume of pancreatic necrosis is noted. A pancreatic necrosectomy is thus performed with packing applied. Haemostasis is achieved at the end.

Clinical pearls

* Pancreatitis usually presents with gastrointestinal symptoms with abdominal pain, vomiting and fever. Less common presentations include skin manifestations, as illustrated in this case.
* If symptoms persist or worsen, early imaging to identify local complications is warranted.

Impress your attending

What is pancreatic panniculitis?

This is a condition characterised by subcutaneous fat necrosis that affects patients with various pancreatic disorders. Treatment is directed at the underlying disease.

Histologically, enzymatic fat necrosis with smudgy ghost shadows of adipocytes with basophilic deposition of calcium salts (saponification) is seen (Figure 7.4).

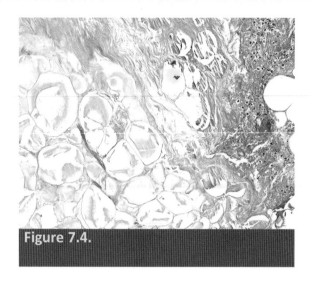

Figure 7.4.

Which pancreatic malignancy is most strongly associated with the development of pancreatic panniculitis?
Acinar cell carcinoma of the pancreas [3].

What is Schmid's triad?

The presence of pancreatic panniculitis, polyarthritis and eosinophilia has been reported to be associated with acinar cell carcinoma of the pancreas and pertains to a poor prognosis.

References

1. Al-Omran M, Albalawi ZH, Tashkandi MF, Al-Ansary LA. Enteral versus parenteral nutrition for acute pancreatitis. *Cochrane Database Syst Rev* 2010; 1: CD002837.
2. Isenmann R, Runzi M, Kron M, *et al.* Prophylactic antibiotic treatment in patients with predicted severe acute pancreatitis: a placebo-controlled, double-blind trial. *Gastroenterology* 2004; 126: 997-1004.
3. Beltraminelli HS, Buechner SA, Häuserman P. Pancreatic panniculitis in a patient with acinar cell cystadenocarcinoma of the pancreas. *Dermatology* 2004; 208: 265-7.

Case 8

History

A 23-year-old lady noted a painful rash over her right shin with a progressive increase in size and discharge over 1 week (Figure 8.1). She also reports a history of generalised malaise, abdominal discomfort and weight loss over the past few months. She denies any history of rheumatological or dermatological diseases.

Physical examination

- Temperature 37.1°C, pulse 72 bpm, BP 115/60mmHg, SaO_2 98-100% on RA.
- Peripheral pulses are strong, with no varicose veins or pigmentation over the gaiter's area (Figure 8.1).
- Hydration is satisfactory.
- Examination of the hands reveals no clubbing and normal-appearing palmar creases.
- Head and neck examination is unremarkable.
- Cardiovascular: HS dual, no murmur.
- Her chest is clear on auscultation.
- Abdominal examination reveals a soft, non-tender abdomen.
- No signs of oedema.

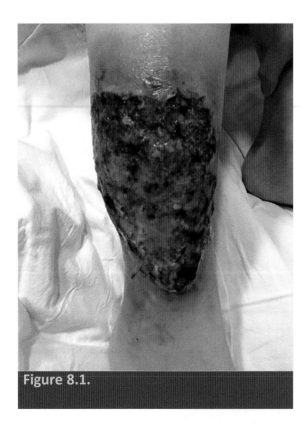

Figure 8.1.

Please describe what you see

There is a deep ulcerating, necrotic lesion with an undermined ulcer edge and bluish border. The surrounding skin is erythematous.

Investigations

- CBC:
    - WBC 9.5 x 10⁹/L;
    - haemoglobin 9.6g/dL;
    - platelets 340 x 10⁹/L.
- ESR 26mm/hr.
- CRP 22.2mg/L.

What is your differential diagnosis?

- Infection:
    - bacterial (i.e. erysipelas, gangrene, late syphilis);
    - mycobacterial;
    - fungal (i.e. sporotrichosis);
    - parasitic;
    - viral (i.e. deep herpetic infections).
- Malignancy:
    - squamous cell carcinoma;
    - basal cell carcinoma;
    - cutaneous T-cell lymphoma.
- Vascular:
    - venous or arterial insufficiency;
    - antiphospholipid syndrome.
- Vasculitis:
    - rheumatoid arthritis;
    - Behçet's disease;
    - Wegener's granulomatosis.
- Drugs (pustular drug eruptions).
- Exogenous tissue injury:
    - factitious panniculitis as part of Munchausen syndrome;
    - insect bites.

- Inflammatory:
  - pyoderma gangrenosum (PG);
  - Sweet's syndrome (acute febrile neutrophilic dermatosis).

What would you do next?

- X-ray of the tibia/fibula for any osteolytic lesions or erosions.
- Wound swabs to exclude infection.
- Biopsy of the lesion to exclude malignancy, infection or cutaneous vasculitis.
- In view of her gastrointestinal symptoms, further work-up for underlying inflammatory bowel disease such as endoscopy or computed tomography (CT) can be considered.

A CT enteroclysis is performed for this lady (Figure 8.2).

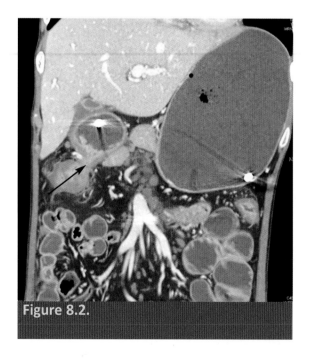

Figure 8.2.

Please describe what you see
A feeding tube is *in situ* with a distended duodenum and stomach. A suspected duodeno-enteric fistula is noted.

What is the most compatible diagnosis?

Pyoderma gangrenosum, likely associated with underlying fistulizing Crohn's disease.

Clinical pearls

* Pyoderma gangrenosum is a neutrophilic dermatosis affecting the skin. It is essentially a diagnosis of exclusion, and ruling out infection is essential as the mainstay of treatment involves immunosuppression.
* The clinical course is variable and it is not related to the activity of the underlying inflammatory bowel disease.

Impress your attending

What are the systemic diseases associated with pyoderma gangrenosum?
Around 50% of patients with PG have underlying inflammatory bowel disease, myeloproliferative disease or rheumatological disease.

The most common underlying disease associated with PG in adults is inflammatory bowel disease (PG has been reported in 1-10% of ulcerative colitis and 0.5-20% of Crohn's disease patients [1]).

How would you manage this patient?
* Local:
    - hydroactive or foam dressings;
    - topical corticosteroids or injection of steroids into the ulcer edge;
    - topical tacrolimus.
* Systemic:
    - corticosteroids +/- minocycline;

- cyclosporin (other immunosuppressives such as azathioprine, tacrolimus, mycofenolate mofetil have also been used);
- biologics such as infliximab. Brooklyn *et al* conducted the only randomised controlled trial to date for the treatment of pyoderma gangrenosum, and showed a clinical improvement when compared with placebo (46% vs. 6%; p = 0.025) [2].

What other extra-intestinal manifestations (EIM) of inflammatory bowel disease do you know of [3]*?*

- Skin:
    - oral aphthous ulcers;
    - Sweet's syndrome;
    - erythema nodosum;
    - pyoderma gangrenosum.
- Eyes:
    - episcleritis;
    - uveitis.
- Joints:
    - Type I (pauciarticular) peripheral arthropathy;
    - Type II (polyarticular) peripheral arthropathy — separate disease course with regard to IBD intestinal activity;
    - axial arthropathy — separate disease course with regard to IBD intestinal activity.

References

1. Lebwohl M, Lebwohl O. Cutaneous manifestations of inflammatory bowel disease. *Inflamm Bowel Dis* 1998; 4: 142-8.
2. Brooklyn TN, Dunnill MG, Shetty A, *et al.* Infliximab for the treatment of pyoderma gangrenosum: a randomised, double blind, placebo controlled trial. *Gut* 2006; 55(4): 505-9.
3. Vavricka SR, Schoepfer A, Scharl M, *et al.* Extraintestinal manifestations of inflammatory bowel disease. *Inflamm Bowel Dis* 2015; 21(8): 1982-92.

Case 9

A 68-year-old lady with a history of hypertension and hypothyroidism presents to the accident and emergency department with a 2-day history of right upper quadrant pain and jaundice. There is no recent travel history.

Physical examination

- Afebrile, pulse 70 bpm, BP 120/65mmHg, SaO_2 98-100% on RA.
- Hydration is satisfactory.
- Examination of the hands reveals no clubbing and normal-appearing palmar creases.
- Head and neck examination is unremarkable.
- Cardiovascular: HS dual, no murmur.
- Her chest is clear on auscultation.
- Abdominal examination reveals a soft abdomen, with mild right upper quadrant tenderness and no other peritoneal signs.
- No signs of oedema.

Investigations

- CBC:
  - WBC 3.5 x 10^9/L;
  - haemoglobin 9.9g/dL;
  - platelets 275 x 10^9/L.
- ALP 661 IU/L.
- Bilirubin 18μmol/L.
- ALT 53 IU/L.
- GGT 1127 IU/L.
- International Normalised Ratio (INR) 1.62.
- Amylase normal.
- CRP normal.
- Anti-HAV IgM, HBsAg, anti-HCV, anti-HEV IgM negative.

What is your differential diagnosis?

- Acute cholangitis.
- Mirizzi syndrome.
- Malignant obstruction.

What further investigations would you arrange?

Imaging studies, i.e. ultrasonography, computed tomography, are required (Figure 9.1).

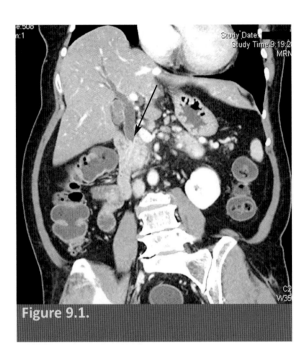

Figure 9.1.

Please describe what you see
A coronal CT scan of the abdomen with contrast. The common bile duct is moderately dilated measuring 1.3cm at the mid portion. It shows an abrupt change of calibre at the pancreatic head level. There is also suspicious diffuse ductal wall thickening at the distal common bile duct. There are no definite intraductal filling defects.

Does this narrow your differential diagnosis?

The most compatible diagnosis is cholangiocarcinoma of the common bile duct.

How would you treat this patient?

A Whipple operation (or pylorus-preserving pancreaticoduodenectomy) for curative resection.

The following is a histological photo of the pancreatic surgical specimen (Figure 9.2).

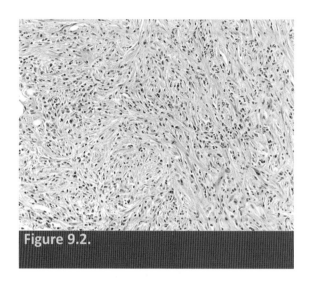

Figure 9.2.

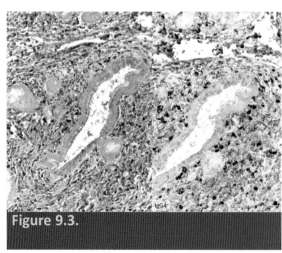

Figure 9.3.

Please describe what you see

There are prominent lymphoplasmacytic infiltrates throughout the pancreas. There are no apparent atypical lymphoid cells. Prominent fibrosis is noted in the surrounding stroma. This lesion extends to the adjacent structures including the common bile duct.

Immunohistochemical studies show scattered plasma cells staining for IgG and some are IgG4 positive (Figure 9.3). Kappa and Lambda stains show no light chain restriction.

Further blood taking for serum IgG4 levels is markedly elevated at 3245g/L.

What is the final diagnosis?

IgG4-related disease (IgG4-RD).

Clinical pearls

- IgG4-related disease is an increasingly recognised disease entity characterised by fibroinflammation and tumour-like lesions in affected organs. It can affect several different organs and can masquerade as malignant tumours, such as in this case.
- This disease is more common in men and in patients older than 50 years of age [1].
- The key histopathological features of this condition [2] include dense lymphoplasmacytic and eosinophilic infiltrates, storiform fibrosis and obliterative phlebitis.

Impress your attending

What organ systems can be affected by IgG4-related disease (Table 9.1 [3])?

Table 9.1. Organ systems affected by IgG4-related disease.

Recognised conditions	Affected organ systems
Mikulicz's syndrome	Salivary and lacrimal glands
Küttner's tumour	Submandibular glands
Riedel's thyroiditis	Thyroid
Eosinophilic angiocentric fibrosis	Orbits and upper respiratory tract
Multifocal fibrosclerosis	Multiple sites
Inflammatory pseudotumour	Multiple sites
Tubulointerstitial nephritis	Kidneys
Periaortitis, inflammatory aortic aneurysm	Major arteries
Retroperitoneal fibrosis	Retroperitoneum

What is the treatment for IgG4-related disease?
- First-line therapy consists of glucocorticoids [4].
- Steroid-sparing agents such as azathioprine, mycophenolate mofetil and methotrexate can be considered for long-term therapy.
- There are case reports suggesting that B-cell depletion with rituximab may be useful in refractory or recurrent cases [5].

Do you know of any new biomarkers under investigation for the use in IgG4-related disease?
Circulating plasmablast counts were shown to be elevated in active IgG4-related disease [6]. The elevation was still present even in patients with normal serum IgG4 concentrations. This may be a potential new biomarker for diagnosis and the monitoring of response to treatment.

References

1. Frulloni L, Lunardi C, Simone R, *et al*. Identification of a novel antibody associated with autoimmune pancreatitis. *N Engl J Med* 2009; 361: 2135-42.
2. Deshpande V, Gupta R, Sainani NI, *et al*. Subclassification of autoimmune pancreatitis: a histologic classification with clinical significance. *Am J Surg Pathol* 2011; 35: 26-35.
3. Stone JH, Zen Y, Deshpande V. IgG4-related disease. *N Engl J Med* 2012; 366(6): 539-51.
4. Kamisawa T, Okazaki K, Kawa S, *et al*. Japanese consensus guidelines for management of autoimmune pancreatitis. III. Treatment and prognosis of AIP. *J Gastroenterol* 2010; 45: 471-7.
5. Khosroshahi A, Carruthers M, Deshpande V, *et al*. Rituximab for the treatment of IgG4-related disease: lessons from ten consecutive patients. *Medicine* (Baltimore) 2012; 91: 57-66.
6. Wallace ZS, Mattoo H, Carruthers M, *et al*. Plasmablasts as a biomarker for IgG4-related disease, independent of serum IgG4 concentrations. *Ann Rheum Dis* 2015; 74(1): 190.

Case 10

History

A 90-year-old chairbound lady from a residence home with a history of dementia presented with a cough and yellowish sputum. She was treated with antibiotics for chest infection by her general practitioner. She subsequently presents with watery diarrhoea, poor oral intake and reduced responsiveness.

Physical examination

- Afebrile, pulse ~100 bpm, BP 63/43mmHg, SaO_2 98-100% on RA.
- Hydration very dry.
- Tired looking, but her GCS is 15/15.
- Examination of the hands reveals no clubbing and normal-appearing palmar creases.
- Head and neck examination is unremarkable.
- Cardiovascular: HS dual, no murmur.
- Her chest is clear on auscultation.
- Abdominal examination reveals a soft abdomen, grossly distended with generalised tenderness and sluggish bowel sounds.
- Per rectal examination: no hematochezia, melaena.
- No signs of oedema.

Investigations

- CBC:
  - WBC 12.2 x 10^9/L;
  - haemoglobin 12.1g/dL;
  - platelets 254 x 10^9/L.
- CRP 31.3mg/L.
- Na^+ 146mmol/L.
- K^+ 2.9mmol/L.
- Creatinine 71μmol/L.
- Albumin 32g/L.
- Other liver function tests are normal.
- CXR: mild right lower lobe haziness. No free gas under the diaphragm.
- AXR (Figure 10.1).

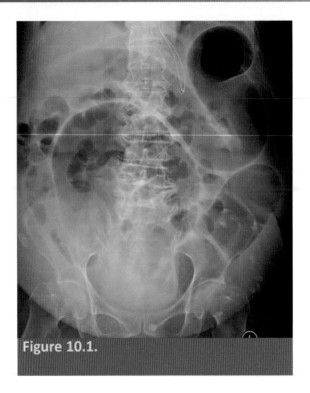

Figure 10.1.

Please describe what you see
There is a dilated transverse colon with a loss of haustra.

What is the likely diagnosis?

Clostridium difficile-associated colitis (CDAD) complicated with toxic megacolon, which is later on confirmed by the detection of *Clostridium difficile* toxin B gene DNA.

How would you manage this patient?

Fluid resuscitation of 2L of normal saline intravenous fluids should be given for her hypovolaemic shock. Her blood pressure responds briskly to the fluid challenge, with a recheck systolic blood pressure of 110mmHg.

Intravenous metronidazole and oral vancomycin should be started.

Close monitoring of symptoms, vital signs and laboratory parameters are required.

Surgical consultation should be sought (in the case of worsening of symptoms and a high risk for perforation).

Clinical pearls

- *Clostridium difficile* is a Gram-positive, anaerobic, spore-forming bacilli found in soil, water, hospital environments and in the gastrointestinal tract of mammals. It is transmitted via the faecal-oral route. The spores are resistant to alcohol and acid [1]. It is a leading cause of nosocomial infection in developed countries.
- The postulated pathogenesis of CDAD involves the disruption of colonic microflora due to the use of antibiotics. With a susceptible gut environment, exposure to *C. difficile* leads to colonisation with the production of cytotoxins, which ultimately lead to pseudomembranous colitis.

Impress your attending

What C. difficile toxins do you know of [2]?
- Toxin A: affects the apical cell membrane leading to cytoskeletal disruption and loosening of the epithelial barrier and disruption of tight junctions.
- Toxin B: affects the basolateral membrane. This is responsible for the virulence of *C. difficile* infection via inducing the release of immunomodulatory mediators.
- Binary toxin.

What is the incidence of Clostridium difficile-associated disease?
Clostridium difficile-associated disease (CDAD) is becoming more common. The incidence has increased from 35.6 to 156.3 per 100,000 population from 1991 to 2003 [3].

What are the risk factors for CDAD?

These include advanced age, recent hospitalisation, resident in long-term care facilities, recent use of antibiotics, and the use of proton pump inhibitors [4].

How would you distinguish between non-severe and severe (fulminant) CDAD (Table 10.1)?

Table 10.1. Distinguishing features of non-severe and severe (fulminant) CDAD [3].

	Non-severe	**Severe**
Symptoms	Watery diarrhoea	May have ileus
	Abdominal pain/cramps	
Signs	Fever	Temperature ≥38.5°C
	Tachycardia	Shock
	Hypovolaemia	Guarding, rebound if perforation
	Abdominal distension	
		Altered mental state
Lab results	Leukocytosis (frequently ≥15 x 10⁹/L)	WCC can be as high as 40 x 10⁹/L
	Deranged RFT (creatinine <1.5x premorbid level)	Deranged RFT (creatinine ≥1.5x premorbid level)
		Hypoalbuminaemia
		Dilated bowels on AXR

How would you manage patients with CDAD (Figures 10.2 and 10.3 [5]?

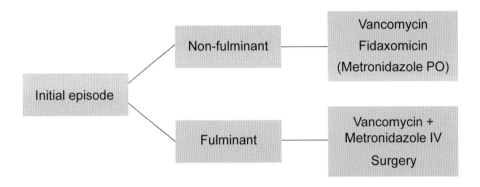

Figure 10.2. An algorithm for managing an initial episode of CDAD.

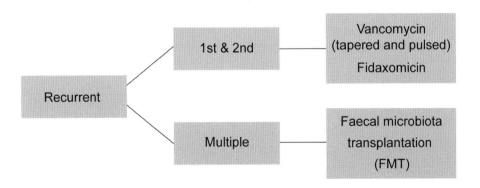

Figure 10.3. An algorithm for managing recurrent CDAD.

Is there any evidence supporting the use of faecal microbiota transplantation (FMT) for recurrent CDAD?

There is a growing body of evidence suggesting that FMT is highly effective for the treatment of recurrent CDAD. In a landmark study in the Netherlands by van Nood *et al* [6], 13 of 16 patients (81%) in the FMT infusion group achieved resolution of *C. difficile*-associated diarrhoea compared with 4 of 13 patients (31%) treated with vancomycin alone and 3 of 13 patients (23%) treated with vancomycin with bowel lavage (p <0.001 for both comparisons with the infusion group). There were no significant differences in adverse events among the three study groups except for mild diarrhoea and abdominal cramping in the infusion group.

References

1. Riggs MM, Sethi AK, Zabarsky TF, *et al.* Asymptomatic carriers are a potential source for transmission of epidemic and non-epidemic *Clostridium difficile* strains among long-term care facility residents. *Clin Infect Dis* 2007; 45(8): 992.

2. Rupnik M, Wilcox MH, Gerding DN. *Clostridium difficile* infection: new developments in epidemiology and pathogenesis. *Nat Rev Microbiol* 2009; 7: 526-36.

3. Pépin J, Valiquette L, Alary ME, *et al. Clostridium difficile*-associated diarrhea in a region of Quebec from 1991 to 2003: a changing pattern of disease severity. *CMAJ* 2004; 171(5): 466-72.

4. Loo VG, Bourgault AM, Poirier L, *et al.* Host and pathogen factors for *Clostridium difficile* infection and colonization. *N Engl J Med* 2011; 365(18): 1693-703.

5. McDonald LC, Gerding DN, Johnson S, *et al.* Clinical practice guidelines for *Clostridium difficile* infection in adults and children: 2017 Update by the Infectious Diseases Society of America (IDSA) and Society for Healthcare Epidemiology of America (SHEA). *Clin Infect Dis* 2018; 66(7): e1-e48.

6. van Nood E, Vrieze A, Nieuwdorp M, *et al.* Duodenal infusion of donor feces for recurrent *Clostridium difficile*. *N Engl J Med* 2013; 368(5): 407-15.

Case 11

History

A 56-year-old gentleman is admitted for severe epigastric pain, tarry stools and generalised malaise. He has a past history of ischaemic heart disease, gout and recent biliary pancreatitis which he underwent endoscopic retrograde cholangiopancreatography for stone removal. He is a non-drinker and takes a COX-2 inhibitor for his joint pain.

Physical examination

- Low-grade fever, pulse 100 bpm, BP 124/69mmHg, SaO_2 97% on RA.
- Hydration is satisfactory.
- Examination of the hands reveals no clubbing and normal-appearing palmar creases.
- Head and neck examination is unremarkable.
- Cardiovascular: HS dual, no murmur.
- His chest is clear on auscultation.
- Abdominal examination reveals mild epigastric discomfort, with no definite mass.
- Per rectal examination: old melaena.
- No signs of oedema.

Investigations

- CBC:
  - WBC 12.2 x 10^9/L;
  - haemoglobin 10.4g/dL dropped to 8.5g/dL;
  - platelets 259 x 10^9/L.
- CXR: grossly clear, with no free gas under the diaphragm.
- Urea normal.
- Amylase 310 IU/L.
- Liver and renal function tests are normal.

What is your differential diagnosis?

- Peptic ulcer bleeding (secondary to NSAIDs).
- Small bowel enteropathy (secondary to NSAIDs).
- Post-ERCP sphincterotomy bleeding.

What would you do next?

- Empirical antibiotics and supportive transfusion should be initiated.

- Oesophagogastroduodenoscopy (OGD):
  - first-look OGD: the ampulla with an existing sphincterotomy is noted next to a peri-ampullary diverticulum. There is no active bleeding;
  - in view of ongoing active bleeding, a second-look OGD is arranged (Figure 11.1).

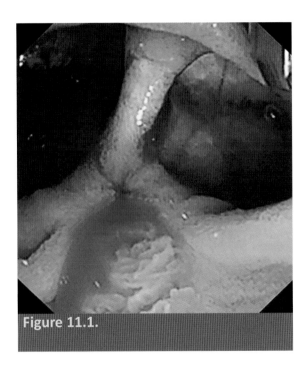

Figure 11.1.

Please describe what you see

Bloody pancreatic juices and red blood are noted oozing from the ampullary orifice.

What is the working diagnosis?

Haemosuccus pancreaticus.

What would you do next?

An urgent angiography should be done to achieve haemostasis. A small pseudoaneurysm arising from a tiny proximal branch of the splenic artery is noted with no active contrast extravasation. Selective embolisation is not successful (Figure 11.2).

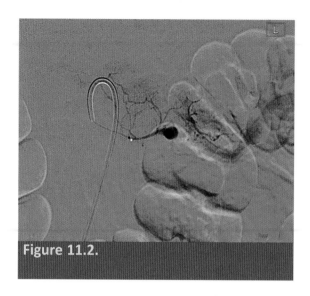

Figure 11.2.

Subsequently, the patient develops haemodynamic instability with a further haemoglobin drop. The surgical team is consulted and a distal pancreatectomy and splenectomy are performed.

Clinical pearls

- Haemosuccus pancreaticus is a rare cause of upper gastrointestinal haemorrhage with bleeding from the pancreatic duct.
- Treatment options include angiographic embolisation and surgery.

Impress your attending

What is the nature of the pain in this condition?
It has been described to be cresendo-decrescendo in nature. This is postulated to be due to the transient blockage of the pancreatic duct from blood clots [1].

What are the causes of haemosuccus pancreaticus [2]?
- 80% of cases are caused by underlying pancreatic disease:
  - chronic pancreatitis;
  - pancreatic tumours;
  - pancreatic ductal stones;
  - complications of procedures;
  - pancreas divisum.
- Around 20% of causes correspond to a vascular anomaly:
  - aneurysms;
  - pseudoaneurysms;
  - arteriovenous malformations.

References

1. Clay R, Farnell M, Lancaster J, *et al.* Hemosuccus pancreaticus. An unusual cause of upper gastrointestinal bleeding. *Ann Surg* 1985; 202(1): 75-9.
2. Vimalraj V, Kannan DG, Sukumar R, *et al.* Haemosuccus pancreaticus: diagnostic and therapeutic challenges. *HPB* 2009; 11: 345-50.

Case 12

History

A 78-year-old smoker was referred to the medical clinic for weight loss of 5kg in the past few months. This was associated with malaise. He denies abdominal pain, yellowing of sclera or tea-coloured urine. He has a history of chronic obstructive pulmonary disease and is an ex-intravenous drug user.

Physical examination

- Afebrile, pulse 68 bpm, BP 122/70mmHg, SaO$_2$ 98-100% on RA.
- Hydration fair, cachexic.
- Examination of the hands reveals no clubbing and normal-appearing palmar creases.
- Head and neck examination is unremarkable.
- Cardiovascular: HS dual, no murmur.
- His chest is clear on auscultation.
- Abdominal examination reveals a soft abdomen, with irregular hepatomegaly ~1-2cm below the right subcostal margin. There is no shifting dullness.
- No signs of oedema.

Investigations

- CBC:
  - WBC 5.7 x 10^9/L;
  - haemoglobin 12.2g/dL;
  - platelets 163 x 10^9/L.
- Bilirubin 10µmol/L.
- ALP 110 IU/L.
- ALT 44 IU/L.
- Alpha-fetoprotein (AFP) 34µg/L.
- Adjusted calcium normal.
- Anti-HCV Ab positive.
- HBsAg negative.

What is your working diagnosis?

In view of a history of intravenous drug use and hepatitis C status, together with the constitutional symptoms, irregular hepatomegaly on palpation and raised AFP, hepatocellular carcinoma (HCC) is an important differential diagnosis. Another differential diagnosis includes liver metastases.

How would you proceed?

A triphasic computed tomography (CT) scan of the liver should be arranged (Figures 12.1-12.3).

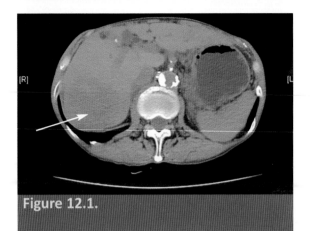

Figure 12.1.

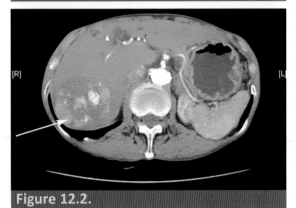

Figure 12.2.

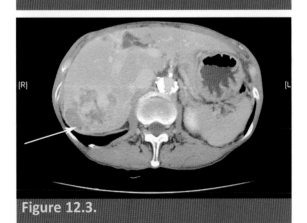

Figure 12.3.

Please describe what you see

Figure 12.1 is a pre-contrast CT film showing a large, vague hypodense lesion at the right posterior segment of the liver. Figure 12.2 demonstrates early arterial enhancement of the lesion. Figure 12.3 shows early washout of contrast. These CT findings are diagnostic of hepatocellular carcinoma (HCC).

What would be the next step of management?

Referral to a multidisciplinary clinic for hepatocellular carcinoma is important.

The following image is acquired after treatment (Figure 12.4).

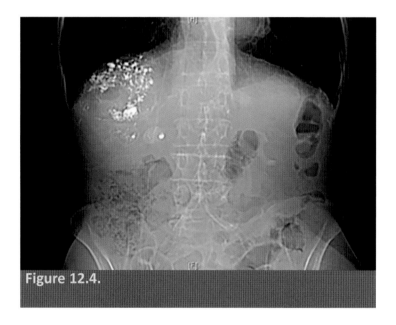

Figure 12.4.

What therapy was given to this patient?

The radio-opaque substance noted in the right upper quadrant is Lipiodol®. This patient underwent transarterial chemoembolisation (TACE).

Clinical pearls

- For subjects with HCC, tumour burden, liver function and performance status of the patient needs to be considered when evaluating treatment options.
- TACE is a non-curative treatment which involves the injection of chemotherapy followed by embolisation of the feeding hepatic artery to achieve tumour necrosis. This therapy is based on the principle that HCCs are highly vascularised and mostly dependent upon the hepatic artery for blood supply.

Impress your attending

What are the risk factors for HCC?
- Cirrhosis (infection with HBV or HCV, alcoholic liver disease, non-alcoholic fatty liver disease [NAFLD], aflatoxin exposure, autoimmune hepatitis and rarer hereditary causes such as hereditary haemochromatosis, Wilson's disease, etc).
- Age.
- Male sex.
- Family history of HCC.

What tests are used as surveillance for HCC in at-risk populations?
- Ultrasound (sensitivity ~65% and specificity of >90%)[1].
- Alpha-fetoprotein (AFP).

Do you know of any newer biomarkers?
Lens culinaris agglutinin-reactive fraction of AFP (AFP-L3) and des-gamma-carboxy prothrombin (DCP) are newer biomarkers that improve

the sensitivity and specificity of detecting early-stage HCC when combined with ultrasound.

How is HCC staged?

There are various systems proposed, with the Barcelona Clinic Liver Cancer (BCLC) Staging System [2] offering the most prognostic information (Figure 12.5 [3]).

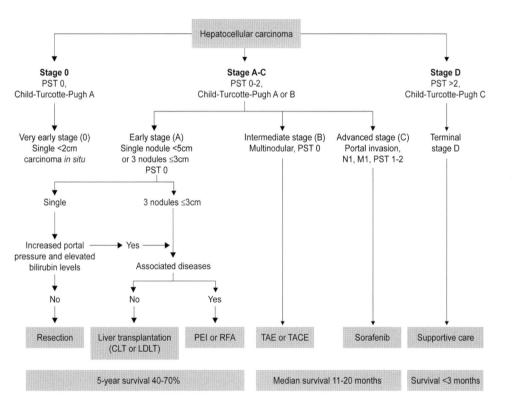

PST: performance status test.
CLT: cadaveric liver transplantation.
LDLT: living donor liver transplantation.
PEI: percutaneous ethanol injection.
RFA: radiofrequency ablation.
TA(C)E: transarterial (chemo)-embolisation.

Figure 12.5. The Barcelona Clinic Liver Cancer (BCLC) Staging System.

In patients with HCC and cirrhosis, which patients are generally deemed suitable for the consideration of liver transplantation?
According to the Milan Criteria [4], a patient is suitable for transplantation if:

- Solitary HCC <5cm.
- Up to three nodules <3cm in size.
- No extrahepatic involvement.
- No vascular invasion.

In well selected cases, the 5-year survival after liver transplantation is up to 75%.

What chemotherapeutic agents are injected during a session of TACE?
Chemotherapy (commonly Adriamycin® or cisplatin) is usually suspended in Lipiodol®. Lipiodol® is selectively retained within the tumour and expands the exposure of the neoplastic cells to chemotherapy. Subsequently, arterial obstruction is achieved by injection of various agents such as Gelfoam®.

What is post-embolisation syndrome?
These are the symptoms that arise from the acute ischaemia of the HCC. They appear in more than 50% of patients receiving TACE. These include:

- Fever.
- Abdominal pain.
- Ileus.

References

1. Singal A, Volk ML, Waljee A, *et al*. Meta-analysis: surveillance with ultrasound for early-stage hepatocellular carcinoma in patients with cirrhosis. *Aliment Pharmacol Ther* 2009; 30: 37-47.

2. Llovet JM, Bru C, Bruix J. Prognosis of hepatocellular carcinoma: the BCLC staging classification. *Semin Liver Dis* 1999; 19: 329-38.
3. Cabibbo G, Latteri F, Antonucci M, Craxì A. Multimodal approaches to the treatment of hepatocellular carcinoma. *Nat Clin Pract Gastroenterol Hepatol* 2009; 6(3): 159-69.
4. Mazzaferro V, Regalia E, Doci R, *et al*. Liver transplantation for the treatment of small hepatocellular carcinomas in patients with cirrhosis. *N Engl J Med* 1996; 334: 693-9.

Case 13

A 62-year-old gentleman is admitted for a chest infection. He has a past history of nasopharyngeal carcinoma and pulmonary tuberculosis. A chest computed tomography scan is performed. An incidental finding of a cystic pancreatic dilatation is noted. He denies any abdominal pain, weight loss or change in bowel habit.

Physical examination

- Afebrile, pulse 80 bpm, BP 115/78mmHg, SaO_2 96% on RA.
- Hydration is satisfactory.
- Examination of the hands reveals no clubbing and normal-appearing palmar creases.
- Head and neck examination is unremarkable.
- Cardiovascular: HS dual, no murmur.
- His chest is clear on auscultation.
- Abdominal examination reveals a soft, non-tender abdomen, with no definite mass palpable.
- No signs of oedema.

Investigations

- CBC:
    - WBC 5.8×10^9/L;
    - haemoglobin 11.8g/dL;
    - platelets 283×10^9/L.
- ALP 138 IU/L.
- ALT 16 IU/L.
- Bilirubin 4µmol/L.
- Amylase 81 IU/L.
- CA 19.9 is 457 kIU/L (reference range is <18).

What would you do next?

A formal CT of the abdomen and pelvis with contrast (Figure 13.1).

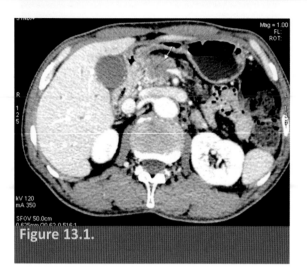

Figure 13.1.

Please describe what you see

A 2.3cm x 2.7cm hypoenhancing solid lesion in the pancreatic head/neck with an irregular border is seen. The overall appearance is suggestive of a pancreatic tumour causing ductal obstruction and parenchymal atrophy.

How would you treat this patient?

In view of his young age and good premorbid condition and features highly suggestive of malignancy on imaging, he should be referred for surgery.

A total pancreatectomy with splenectomy is performed which shows a 4cm infiltrative tumour at the pancreatic head with local invasion at the portal vein/superior mesenteric vein junction. There are enlarged lymph nodes at the common hepatic artery, coeliac trunk and aortocaval window. There is no liver or peritoneal metastasis.

Final histology shows a moderately differentiated adenocarcinoma of the head of the pancreas with a maximum dimension of 4cm.

Clinical pearls

- Early pancreatic cancer can be elusive. When signs and symptoms such as abdominal pain, jaundice, steatorrhoea, gastrointestinal bleeding, weight loss develop, the disease has likely progressed to an advanced stage. A high index of suspicion is warranted.
- Risk factors include [1]:
  - smoking;
  - obesity;
  - diabetes;
  - chronic pancreatitis (controversial);
  - family history.

Impress your attending

What are the limitations of CA 19-9?
CA stands for carbohydrate antigen or cancer antigen.

It is not specific for pancreatic adenocarcinoma, and may be falsely elevated in conditions such as cholestasis. In addition, patients with a negative Lewis antigen A or B are unable to synthesize CA 19-9, leading to undetectable levels.

Do you know of any poor prognostic factors for pancreatic cancer?
- High tumour grade.
- Large tumour.
- Positive margins of resection.
- Lymph node metastases.
- High levels of CA 19-9.

What is the prognosis of pancreatic adenocarcinoma?
In general the prognosis is poor with overall 5-year survival of around 6%. For local disease the 5-year survival is approximately 24% [2].

What would be the choice of chemotherapy after curative resection?

According to the CONKO-001 trial [3], among patients with macroscopic complete removal of pancreatic cancer, the use of adjuvant gemcitabine for 6 months compared with observation alone resulted in increased overall survival as well as disease-free survival.

References

1. Hassan MM, Bondy ML, Wolff RA, *et al*. Risk factors for pancreatic cancer: case control study. *Am J Gastroenterol* 2007; 102: 2696-707.
2. American Cancer Society. Cancer facts and figures, 2014.
3. Oettle H, Neuhaus P, Hochhaus A, *et al*. Adjuvant chemotherapy with gemcitabine and long-term outcomes among patients with resected pancreatic cancer: the CONKO-001 randomized trial. *JAMA* 2013; 310(14): 1473-81.

Case 14

A 60-year-old lady with a history of neurofibromatosis, mechanical mitral valve replacement and atrial fibrillation on warfarin developed sudden onset postural dizziness upon getting out of bed. She subsequently passed a large amount of tarry stools. There was no haematemesis or coffee ground vomiting. She has good compliance with warfarin and denies any over-the-counter medications.

Physical examination

- Afebrile, pulse 110 bpm, BP 78/42mmHg, SaO_2 98% on RA.
- Conjunctival pallor.
- Examination of the hands reveals no clubbing and normal-appearing palmar creases.
- Head and neck examination is unremarkable.
- Cardiovascular: HS dual, mechanical 1st heart sound.
- Her chest is clear on auscultation.
- Abdominal examination reveals a soft, non-tender abdomen, with no definite mass palpable.
- Per rectal exam: fresh melaena.
- No signs of oedema.

Investigations

- CBC:
  - WBC 13.8 x 10^9/L;
  - haemoglobin 3.6g/dL ← 6.8g/dL ← 10g/dL (baseline);
  - platelets 441 x 10^9/L.
- Urea 15.3mmol/L.
- Creatinine 123µmol/L.
- INR 3.89.
- Liver function tests are grossly normal.
- CXR: no free gas under the diaphragm.
- ECG: sinus tachycardia with a rate around 110 to 120 bpm. No acute ST/T wave changes.

How would you manage this lady?

- Crystalloid fluid resuscitation and blood transfusion.
- Correct the INR with vitamin K and fresh frozen plasma.
- Urgent oesophagogastroduodenoscopy (OGD): a 1.2cm ulcerated submucosal mass next to the ampulla is seen.

What is your differential diagnosis for the mass?

- Gastrointestinal stromal tumour (GIST).
- Neuroendocrine tumour.
- Lymphoma.
- Pancreatic rest.
- Neurofibroma.

What imaging test would you order next?

Computed tomography of the abdomen and pelvis (Figures 14.1 and 14.2).

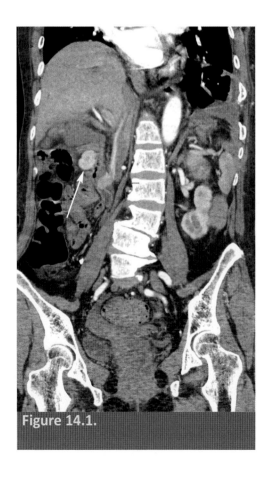

Figure 14.1.

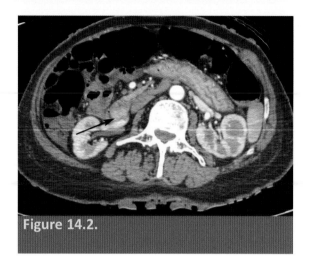

Figure 14.2.

Please describe what you see

An arterial enhancing lesion in D2 without features of intestinal obstruction is noted. There are no features suggestive of metastases.

What further investigations would you request?

An endoscopic ultrasound (Figure 14.3).

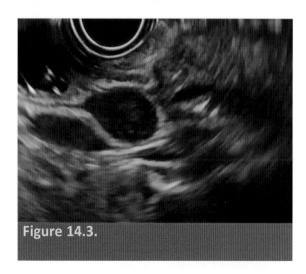

Figure 14.3.

Please describe what you see
At the periampullary region, a well defined, ulcerated submucosal hypoechoic mass is noted. It has a dumbbell-shaped appearance and is connected to the muscularis propria.

What is your diagnosis?

The dumbbell-shaped appearance and the lesion arising from the muscularis propria is more suggestive of GIST.

What would be your next step?

The surgical team should be consulted for resection of the tumour in view of a very high risk of rebleeding if anticoagulation is resumed without definitive treatment.

Local excision of the lesion is done with the subsequent pathological specimen confirming the diagnosis of GIST.

Clinical pearls

- GISTs are uncommon mesenchymal tumours thought to arise from the interstitial cells of Cajal.
- The majority of GISTs are found in the stomach, with many of the smaller-sized lesions found incidentally during endoscopic examination.

Impress your attending

What do you know about the genetics of neurofibromatosis Type 1?
The disease is caused by a mutation on a gene on chromosome 17. It is an autosomal dominant disease, but most cases arise from de novo mutations.

What are the gastrointestinal manifestations of neurofibromatosis Type 1 [1]?

- Neurogenic neoplasms:
  - solitary, plexiform, diffuse mucosal/submucosal neurofibromatosis;
  - gangliocytic paraganglioma.
- Interstitial cell of Cajal lesions:
  - gastrointestinal stromal tumours;
  - interstitial cell of Cajal hyperplasia.
- Neuroendocrine tumours:
  - carcinoid tumour;
  - periampullary somatostatinoma;
  - other neuroendocrine tumours such as insulinomas or gastrinomas.

How would you treat GISTs [2]?

- Localised:
  - if size 2cm or larger, surgical excision;
  - smaller lesions can be excised or closely monitored by endoscopy every 6-12 months.
- Metastatic:
  - first-line: imatinib [3] (tyrosine kinase inhibitor);
  - second-line: sunitinib [4] (tyrosine kinase inhibitor);
  - third-line: regorafenib [5] (multi-kinase inhibitor).

What are good prognostic factors for GIST recurrence after surgery [6]?

These include a smaller tumour size (<2cm), low mitotic count (≤5 per 5mm^2), gastric site of the tumour, and absence of tumour rupture before or during surgery.

Is there a role for adjuvant imatinib?

According to a study by Joensuu et al [7], in patients with operable GISTs and positive KIT or PDGFRA mutation, 3 years compared with 1 year of adjuvant imatinib therapy is associated with longer recurrence-free survival (5-year RFS, 65.6% vs. 47.9%, respectively) and longer overall survival (5-year survival 92% vs. 81.7%, respectively).

How would you decide the timing of resumption of anticoagulation?

The risk of thromboembolic events must be balanced against the risk of bleeding. When facing life-threatening bleeding, full reversal of anticoagulation is warranted even in this setting. Early definitive treatment of the GI bleeding

(GIB) is essential to facilitate the early reintroduction of anticoagulation for prophylaxis against thromboembolic events in high-risk patients.

In a retrospective cohort study of 1329 patients who developed GIB while on anticoagulation for atrial fibrillation, warfarin was restarted in 653 cases (49.1%). Restarting warfarin was associated with decreased thromboembolism and reduced mortality but not recurrent GIB. When stratified by the duration of warfarin interruption, restarting warfarin after 7 days may be beneficial as compared to resuming after 30 days of interruption [8]. The decreased risk of thromboembolism is likely to be even more pronounced in patients with valve replacement.

References

1. Agaimy A, Vassos N, Croner RS. Gastrointestinal manifestations of neurofibromatosis type 1 (Recklinghausen's disease): clinico-pathological spectrum with pathogenetic considerations. *Int J Clin Exp Pathol* 2012; 5(9): 852-62.
2. National Comprehensive Cancer Network. Clinical practice guidelines in oncology: soft tissue sarcoma. Version 2.2014.
3. Verweij J, Casali PG, Zalcberg J, *et al*, for the EORTC Soft Tissue and Bone Sarcoma Group, the Italian Sarcoma Group, and the Australasian Gastrointestinal Trials Group. Progression-free survival in gastrointestinal stromal tumours with high-dose imatinib: randomised trial. *Lancet* 2004; 364: 1127-34.
4. Demetri GD, van Oosterom AT, Garrett CR, *et al*. Efficacy and safety of sunitinib in patients with advanced gastrointestinal stromal tumour after failure of imatinib: a randomised controlled trial. *Lancet* 2006; 368: 1329-38.
5. Demetri GD, Reichardt P, Kang YN, *et al*. Efficacy and safety of regorafenib for advanced gastrointestinal stromal tumours after failure of imatinib and sunitinib (GRID): an international, multicentre, randomised, placebo-controlled, phase 3 trial. *Lancet* 2013; 381: 295-302.
6. Joensuu H. Risk stratification of patients diagnosed with gastrointestinal stromal tumor. *Hum Pathol* 2008; 39: 1411-9.
7. Joensuu H, Eriksson M, Sundby Hall K, *et al*. One vs. three years of adjuvant imatinib for operable gastrointestinal stromal tumor: a randomized trial. *JAMA* 2012; 307(12): 1265-72.
8. Qureshi W, Mittal C, Patsias I, *et al*. Restarting anticoagulation and outcomes after major gastrointestinal bleeding in atrial fibrillation. *Am J Cardiol* 2014; 113(4): 662-8.

Case 15

History

A 56-year-old lady with iron deficiency anaemia had an upper gastrointestinal endoscopy and colonoscopy, both of which were normal. She has been referred to the specialist outpatient clinic with symptoms of increasing abdominal cramps and vomiting over the past few months.

Physical examination

- Afebrile, pulse 90 bpm, BP 120/80mmHg, SaO_2 98-100% on RA.
- Hydration status good.
- Examination of the hands reveals no clubbing and normal-appearing palmar creases.
- Head and neck examination is unremarkable.
- Cardiovascular: HS dual, no murmur.
- Her chest is clear on auscultation.
- Abdominal examination reveals a soft, non-tender abdomen, with no definite mass, and bowel sounds are normal.
- Per rectal exam: yellowish stools only.
- No signs of oedema.

Investigations

- CBC:
  - WBC 3.9×10^9/L;
  - haemoglobin 11g/dL (microcytic hypochromic McHc);
  - platelets 263×10^9/L.
- Liver function tests are normal.
- Renal function tests are normal.
- Amylase normal
- Bone profile is normal.
- CRP normal.
- Preliminary abdominal and chest X-rays are normal.

What would you do next?

In view of her iron deficiency anaemia and progressive symptoms, small bowel investigations should be arranged.

The options for small bowel investigations include:

- Capsule endoscopy.
- Deep enteroscopy (push enteroscopy, single-balloon-assisted enteroscopy, double-balloon enteroscopy, etc.).
- Computed tomography enteroclysis or enterography (CTE); or magnetic resonance enteroclysis or enterography (MRE).

This patient has a CT enterography (Figures 15.1 and 15.2).

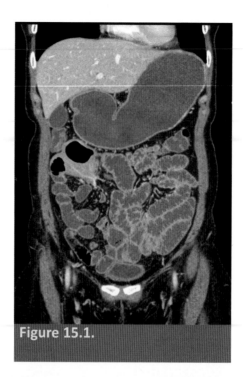

Figure 15.1.

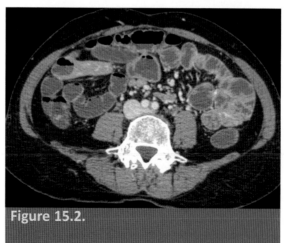

Figure 15.2.

Please describe what you see

A segment of focal small bowel wall thickening is noted at the proximal to mid ileum with stenosis causing partial obstruction, mesenteric thickening and enlarged mesenteric lymph nodes. This was suspicious of infiltrative disease.

What is your differential diagnosis?

- Neoplasm:
  - adenocarcinoma;
  - lymphoma;
  - carcinoid tumour.
- Infection:
  - tuberculosis.

How would you proceed?

An histological specimen is needed for definitive diagnosis. A double-balloon enteroscopy is performed (Figure 15.3).

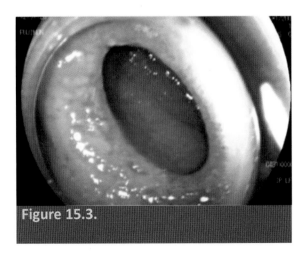

Figure 15.3.

Please describe what you see

An isolated short segment stricture is noted, with some scarring likely from a healed ulcer. Multiple biopsies are taken which are non-diagnostic.

What would you do next?

In view of suspected malignancy, partial intestinal obstruction and negative biopsy findings, surgical resection would be warranted both for diagnostic and therapeutic purposes. A laparoscopic small bowel resection is performed with 15cm of small bowel removed. Figure 15.4 shows the histology specimens below.

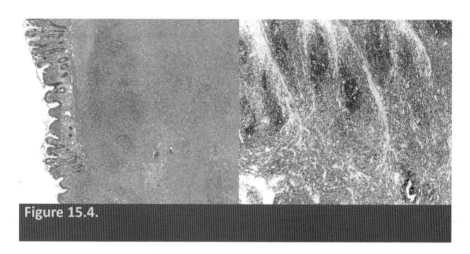

Figure 15.4.

Please describe what you see
A full-thickness infiltration of small bowel by atypical small lymphoid cells with no high-grade component and a clear margin. Tumour cells are CD20+, CD3-, CD5-, CD10-, cyclin D1-, Ki67 ~20%.

What is your final diagnosis?

Extranodal marginal zone lymphoma of mucosa-associated lymphoid tissue (MALT).

Clinical pearls

- With improvements in technology, the small bowel is now more easily assessed by various diagnostic modalities.

- The choice of modality needs to be individualised according to different factors as tabulated below (Table 15.1 [1, 2]).

Table 15.1. Comparison of various modalities in the assessment of the small bowel.

	CTE	MRE	Capsule endoscopy	Enteroscopy (balloon-assisted)
Pros	Simultaneous evaluation of intramural and extramural small bowel disease	Simultaneous evaluation of intramural and extramural small bowel disease	Direct luminal visualisation	Direct luminal visualisation
			Minimally-invasive	Possibility for therapeutic intervention
	Non-invasive	Non-invasive		
				Able to obtain biopsy
Cons	May need nasojejunal tube for enteral contrast with potential discomfort	May need nasojejunal tube for enteral contrast with potential discomfort	Incomplete small bowel visualisation	Requires expertise
				Invasive (potential prolonged duration of procedure and increased amount of sedation) with risks of infection, bleeding, perforation, and pancreatitis shown in some studies
			No manoeuvrability	
	Contrast nephropathy	Risk of NSF in renal failure	Risk of capsule impaction	
	Radiation exposure	Cost and availability	No therapeutic intervention and unable to obtain biopsies	
	No therapeutic intervention and unable to obtain biopsies	No therapeutic intervention and unable to obtain biopsies		

NSF: nephrogenic systemic fibrosis.

Impress your attending

What is the postulated pathogenesis of extranodal marginal zone lymphoma of MALT (MALT lymphoma)?

MALT lymphoma is thought to arise in organs such as the stomach, intestine, lungs, salivary glands, ocular adnexa, etc. that normally lack lymphoid tissue but have accumulated B-cells in response to chronic inflammatory or infective processes [3].

What are the possible aetiologies for the development of gastric and small bowel lymphoma?

Helicobacter pylori (HP) infection has been postulated to cause gastric MALT lymphoma [4].

It has also been shown that *Campylobacter jejuni* is associated with immunoproliferative small intestinal disease [5].

What are the latest developments in the treatment of MALT lymphoma [3]?

For gastric MALT lymphoma, HP eradication may cure early-stage disease.

Radiotherapy may be useful in early-stage gastric MALT lymphoma without evidence of HP infection, persistent gastric MALT lymphoma after antibiotics, or most non-gastric MALT lymphomas.

Combination therapy with rituximab and chlorambucil for patients with persistent gastric MALT lymphoma after antibiotics, or in non-gastric MALT lymphomas, was shown to have significantly better 5-year event-free survival (68% vs. 50%; $p = 0.002$) and a higher complete remission rate in a randomised study by the International Extranodal Lymphoma Study Group published in 2013. However, no statistical significance for progression-free survival and 5-year overall survival was found [6].

References

1. Aktas H, Mensink PB. Small bowel diagnostics: current place of small bowel endoscopy. *Best Practice & Research Clinical Gastroenterology* 2012; 26: 209-20.
2. Pennazio M, Spada C, Eliakim R, *et al*. Small-bowel capsule endoscopy and device-assisted enteroscopy for diagnosis and treatment of small-bowel disorders: European Society of Gastrointestinal Endoscopy (ESGE) Clinical Guideline. *Endoscopy* 2015; 47(04): 352-86.
3. Zinzani PL. The many faces of marginal zone lymphoma. *Hematology Am Soc Hematol Educ Program* 2012; 2012: 426-32.
4. O'Rourke JL. Gene expression profiling in *Helicobacter*-induced MALT lymphoma with reference to antigen drive and protective immunization. *J Gastroenterol Hepatol* 2008; 23(Suppl 2): S151-6.
5. Lecuit M, Abachin E, Martin A, *et al*. Immunoproliferative small intestinal disease associated with *Campylobacter jejuni*. *N Engl J Med* 2004; 350(3): 239-48.
6. Zucca E, Conconi A, Laszlo D, *et al*. Addition of rituximab to chlorambucil produces superior event-free survival in the treatment of patients with extranodal marginal-zone B-cell lymphoma: 5-year analysis of the IELSG-19 randomized study. *J Clin Oncol* 2013; 31(5): 565-72.

Case 16

A 52-year-old lady with a past history of thyroiditis presents with a 6-month history of left lower abdominal pain. There are no constitutional symptoms, change in bowel habit, or rectal bleeding. She is a non-drinker.

Physical examination

- Afebrile, pulse 80 bpm, BP 120/80mmHg, SaO_2 98-100% on RA.
- Hydration is satisfactory.
- Examination of the hands reveals no clubbing and normal-appearing palmar creases.
- Head and neck examination is unremarkable.
- Cardiovascular: HS dual, no murmur.
- Her chest is clear on auscultation.
- Abdominal examination reveals a soft, non-tender abdomen, with no peritoneal signs.
- No signs of oedema.

Investigations

- CBC:
  - WBC 4.7 x 10^9/L;
  - haemoglobin 12g/dL;
  - platelets 177 x 10^9/L.

A computed tomography scan of her abdomen is performed (Figure 16.1).

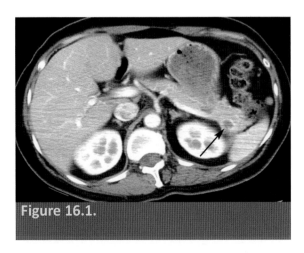

Figure 16.1.

Please describe what you see
There is a cystic lesion with rim enhancement at the tail of the pancreas.

What is your differential diagnosis?

- Non-neoplastic lesion:
  - pseudocyst (accounts for up to 30% of all pancreatic cystic lesions, up to 50% in patients with a history of pancreatitis);
  - true cyst;
  - retention cyst;
  - lymphoepithelial cyst;
  - mucinous non-neoplastic cyst.
- Neoplastic lesion (accounting for ~10-15% of pancreatic cysts):
  - serous cystic neoplasm (SCN);
  - mucinous cystic neoplasm (MCN);
  - intraductal papillary mucinous neoplasm (IPMN):
    - main duct;
    - branch duct;
  - solid pseudopapillary tumour (SPT);
  - cystic pancreatic neuroendocrine tumour (NET);
  - cystic pancreatic ductal adenocarcinoma (PDAC)(cystic degeneration of the tumour).

What further investigations would you arrange?

An endoscopic ultrasound should be arranged for further delineation (Figure 16.2).

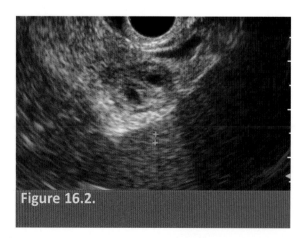

Figure 16.2.

Please describe what you see

A well defined cystic hypoechoic lesion is noted. Fine needle aspiration of the lesion is not done as there is no safe window due to traversing of splenic vessels.

How would you proceed?

In view of uncertainty of the nature of the pancreatic lesion, surgery should be considered for diagnostic and treatment purposes.

A distal pancreatectomy with splenectomy is performed. Histological images are shown below (Figures 16.3 and 16.4).

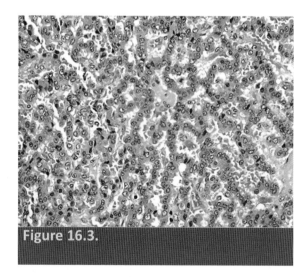

Figure 16.3.

Please describe what you see

The tumour is composed of interconnecting cords and ribbons of tumour cells. The tumour cells are uniform polygonal cells with fine chromatin and a moderate amount of eosinophilic cytoplasm.

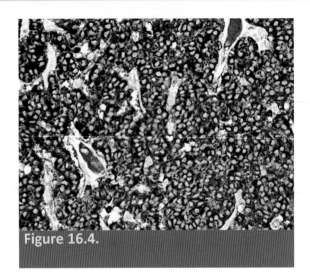

Figure 16.4.

Please describe what you see

The tumour cells are diffusely immunoreactive to a neuroendocrine marker (chromogranin).

What is your final diagnosis?

Neuroendocrine tumour (glucagonoma).

Clinical pearls

- Neuroendocrine tumours (NETs) can either be functional or non-functional. A functional glucagonoma has excessive glucagon secretion and may present as a distinct clinical syndrome with glucose intolerance, weight loss, and a characteristic rash called necrolytic migratory erythema (NME).
- Non-functional tumours usually present as incidental findings on imaging, or present with abdominal pain and/or obstructive symptoms due to their size.

- The diagnosis is supported by elevation in the levels of serum glucagon, but definitive diagnosis requires histopathological assessment of tissue samples obtained from biopsy or surgical specimens.
- Staging and localisation is usually done by somatostatin receptor scintigraphy or positron emission tomography computed tomography (PET-CT), preferably with a dual tracer (dual tracer PET/CT).

Impress your attending

What cells are responsible for endocrine function in the pancreas?

The islets of Langerhans are cell clusters in the pancreas that are responsible for endocrine function. There are four main types of cells:

- Alpha cells — glucagon secretion.
- Beta cells — insulin secretion (most abundant).
- Gamma cells — pancreatic polypeptide secretion.
- Delta cells — somatostatin secretion.

More recently, a fifth type of cell has been identified, now known as epsilon cells which secrete ghrelin [1].

What are the syndromes related to this disease?

Multiple endocrine neoplasia Type 1 (MEN1) is a genetic syndrome associated with the development of parathyroid adenomas, pituitary adenomas and pancreatic islet cell tumours.

How are neuroendocrine tumours graded?

According to the World Health Organization (WHO) classification, NETs can have three grades, taking into account the Ki-67 index and mitotic count per 10 high-power field [2].

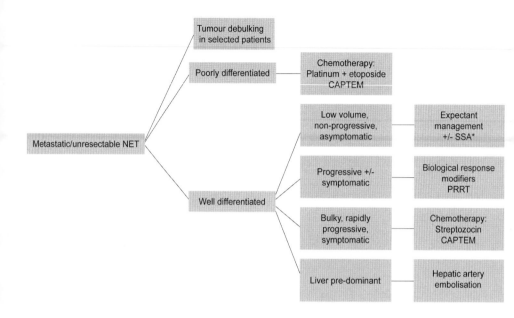

*: more useful for non-pancreatic NETs.

CAPTEM: capecitabine + temozolomide.

SSA: somatostatin analogues.

A recent study published in 2014 using hormonal therapy (lanreotide) in metastatic enteropancreatic neuroendocrine tumours showed a strong anti-proliferative response with prolonged progression-free survival compared with placebo, but not overall survival [4].

PRRT: peptide receptor radionuclide therapy.

In the NETTER-1 phase 3 trial, the use of ^{177}Lu-Dotatate resulted in markedly longer progression-free survival and a significantly higher response rate than high-dose octreotide LAR in patients with advanced midgut neuroendocrine tumours [5].

Figure 16.5. An algorithm for managing metastatic/unresectable neuroendocrine tumours.

What are the treatment options for neuroendocrine tumours?
- Locoregional and resectable → endoscopic resection/surgery.
- Metastatic/unresectable → follow the algorithm on the facing page (Figure 16.5 [3]).

References

1. Assmann A, Hinault C, Kulkarni RN. Growth factor control of pancreatic islet regeneration and function. *Pediatric Diabetes* 2009; 10: 14-32.
2. Bosman FT, Carneiro F, Hruban R, Theise N. WHO Classification of Tumours of the Digestive System, 4th ed. International Agency for Research on Cancer (IARC), Lyon, 2010.
3. Kunz PL. Carcinoid and neuroendocrine tumors: building on success. *J Clin Oncol* 2015; 33(16): 1855-63.
4. Caplin ME, Pavel M, Cwikla JB, *et al*; CLARINET Investigators. Lanreotide in metastatic enteropancreatic neuroendocrine tumors. *N Engl J Med* 2014; 371(3): 224-33.
5. Strosberg J, El-Haddad G, Wolin E, *et al*; NETTER-1 Trial Investigators. Phase 3 trial of ^{177}Lu-Dotatate for midgut neuroendocrine tumors. *N Engl J Med* 2017; 376(2): 125-35.

Case 17

History

A 62-year-old lady with good past health presents with jaundice and tea-coloured urine. She denies abdominal pain or fever. She is a non-drinker with no history of intravenous drug abuse. She has taken some Chinese herbal drink previously but denies any other over-the-counter medications in the recent few weeks.

Physical examination

- Afebrile, pulse 71 bpm, BP 124/60mmHg, SaO_2 98% on RA.
- Hydration is satisfactory.
- Examination of the hands reveals no clubbing and normal-appearing palmar creases.
- Head and neck examination is unremarkable.
- Cardiovascular: HS dual, no murmur.
- Her chest is clear on auscultation.
- Abdominal examination reveals a soft, non-tender abdomen, with no distension.
- GCS 15/15.
- No focal neurology.
- No flapping tremor.
- No signs of oedema.

Investigations

- CBC:
  - WBC 5×10^9/L;
  - haemoglobin 14g/dL;
  - platelets 243×10^9/L.
- Bilirubin 493µmol/L.
- ALP 193 IU/L.
- ALT 1560 IU/L.
- INR 1.38.
- AFP 5µg/L.
- Albumin 29g/L.
- Globulin 30g/L.

What is your differential diagnosis?

- Viral hepatitis.
- Drug-induced liver injury.
- Autoimmune diseases.
- Wilson's disease (consider genetic disorders in younger individuals).

What other investigations would you perform?

Further blood tests, including hepatitis serology (for hepatitis A, E, B, C), immunoglobulin pattern and autoimmune markers (anti-nuclear antibody, anti-smooth muscle antibody, anti-mitochondrial antibody are useful for elucidating the cause of hepatitis). All the results come back as negative.

Ultrasound shows no focal hepatic lesions.

The traditional Chinese herbal formula is reviewed by the toxicology team but no obvious hepatotoxic agent could be identified.

How would you proceed?

A liver biopsy is warranted in view of diagnostic uncertainty. Histopathological images are shown below (Figures 17.1 and 17.2).

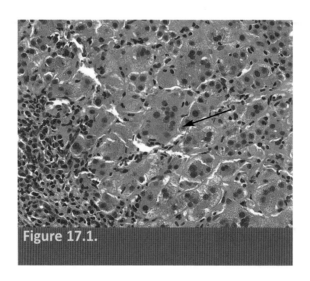

Figure 17.1.

Please describe what you see
A multinucleated hepatocyte (syncytial giant cell) is present.

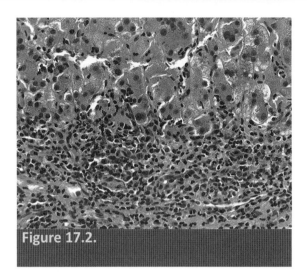

Figure 17.2.

Please describe what you see

Prominent interface hepatitis. There is presence of portal plasma cell infiltrates, marked interface hepatitis and emperipolesis. Some scattered multinucleated giant hepatocytes are identified.

What is the likely diagnosis?

The likely diagnosis is autoimmune hepatitis (AIH) given the typical histological features.

Clinical pearls

- Autoimmune hepatitis (AIH) is an inflammatory condition likely caused by the exposure to environmental triggers in a genetically susceptible individual. Treatment can prevent cirrhosis and improve survival.
- Various criteria have been developed throughout the years to diagnose this condition. Individual factors that have been proposed include female sex, transaminitis, raised serum globulins, positivity of

auto-antibodies (such as anti-nuclear antibodies, anti-smooth muscle antibodies, anti-liver-kidney microsomal antibodies), typical histopathological features on liver biopsy, other associated autoimmune disease, and HLA DR3 or DR4 status.

Modified criteria have been proposed as below (Table 17.1) [1].

Table 17.1. Proposed simplified criteria for autoimmune hepatitis (AIH).

Variable	Cut-off	Points
ANA or ASMA	≥1:40	1
ANA or ASMA	≥1:80	2*
or anti-LKM	≥1:40	2*
or SLA	Positive	2*
IgG	> Upper normal limit	1
	> 1.1 times upper normal limit	2
Liver histology	Compatible with AIH	1
	Typical AIH	2
Absence of viral hepatitis	Yes	2

≥6: probable AIH; ≥7: definite AIH.
* Addition of points achieved for all autoantibodies (maximum, 2 points).
ANA: anti-nuclear antibody.
ASMA: anti-smooth muscle antibody.
anti-LKM: anti-liver-kidney microsomal-1 antibody.
SLA: anti-soluble liver antigen antibody.
IgG: immunoglobulin G.

Impress your attending

What are the types of AIH (Table 17.2) [2]*?*

Table 17.2. Types of AIH.	Type 1	Type 2
Age	All ages	Usually childhood and young adulthood
Clinical phenotype	Variable	Generally severe
Autoantibodies	Anti-nuclear antibody Anti-smooth muscle antibody Others: anti-actin antibody, anti-soluble liver antigen or anti-liver-pancreas antigen antibody	Anti-liver-kidney microsomal antibody Anti-liver-cytosol antibody
Implicated antigenic target	Asialoglycoprotein receptor	Cytochrome p450 2D6
Treatment failure	Rare	More common
Relapse after drug withdrawal	Variable	More common
Need for long-term maintenance	Variable	Almost in all cases

Which histopathological features are typical of AIH?

- Plasma cell infiltrates.
- Interface hepatitis.
- Bridging fibrosis and cirrhosis.

Management of this condition

Immunosuppressants

Induction treatment with corticosteroids, with maintenance of remission with steroid-sparing agents such as azathioprine are the mainstay of therapy. Other agents such as cyclosporine or mycophenolate mofetil may be used if the patient's response is inadequate.

Screening for malignancy

Hepatobiliary and lymphomatous neoplasms are frequent in long-term follow-up in patients with AIH [3]. Screening in cirrhotic patients for hepatocellular carcinoma is warranted.

What is post-infantile giant cell hepatitis?

It is a defined as hepatitis in adults with extensive hepatocyte multi-nucleation. It is rare and is purely a descriptive term that does not have any implications for the aetiology of the hepatitis [4]. It is postulated to arise either from hepatocyte nuclear proliferation that is not followed by cell division, or the fusion of mononuclear hepatocytes [5].

How long should immunosuppressants be given in patients with AIH?

According to the American Association for the Study of Liver Diseases (AASLD) practice guidelines [6], patients should be in biochemical remission for at least 24 months while on therapy before consideration of stopping immunosuppression. A gradual, well-monitored dose reduction over a 6-week period of close surveillance is recommended. However, relapse occurs in approximately 80% of patients who enter remission.

References

1. Hennes EM, Zeniya M, Czaja AJ, *et al.* Simplified criteria for the diagnosis of autoimmune hepatitis. *Hepatology* 2008; 48: 169-76.
2. Heneghan MA, Yeoman AD, Verma S. Autoimmune hepatitis. *Lancet* 2013; 382(9902): 1433-44.
3. Werner M, Almer S, Prytz H, *et al.* Hepatic and extrahepatic malignancies in autoimmune hepatitis: a long-term follow-up in 473 Swedish patients. *J Hepatol* 2009; 50: 388-93.
4. Johnson SJ, Mathew J, MacSween RNM, *et al.* Post-infantile giant cell hepatitis: histological and immunohistochemical study. *J Clin Pathol* 1994; 47(11): 1022-7.
5. Devaney K, Goodman ZD, Ishak KG. Postinfantile giant-cell transformation in hepatitis. *Hepatology* 1992; 16(2): 327-33.
6. Manns MP, Czaja AJ, Gorham JD, *et al*; for the American Association for the Study of Liver Diseases. Diagnosis and management of autoimmune hepatitis. *Hepatology* 2010; 51(6): 2193-213.

Case 18

A 61-year-old postmenopausal lady with a past history of diabetic nephropathy was referred for anaemia. She presents with malaise and shortness of breath. Her haemoglobin is 7g/dL only. She denies symptoms of gastrointestinal bleeding or other bleeding diatheses.

Physical examination

- Afebrile, pulse 95 bpm, BP 114/78mmHg, SaO_2 98-100% on RA.
- Pallor, hydration fair.
- Examination of the hands reveals no clubbing and normal-appearing palmar creases.
- Head and neck examination is unremarkable.
- Cardiovascular: HS dual, no murmur.
- Her chest is clear on auscultation.
- Abdominal examination reveals a soft, non-tender abdomen.
- PR: no melaena.
- No signs of oedema.

Investigations

- CBC:
  - WBC 5 x 10^9/L;
  - haemoglobin 7.3g/dL (microcytic hypochromic);
  - platelets 190 x 10^9/L.
- Urea 25mmol/L.
- Creatinine 400μmol/L.
- Clotting profile is normal.
- Fe 4μmol/L, TIBC 52μmol/L, Fe saturation 7%.

How would you proceed?

This lady has iron deficiency anaemia. In general, chronic blood loss from the gastrointestinal tract or gynaecological causes (less likely in this case) should be considered. An oesophagogastroduodenoscopy (OGD) is performed (Figure 18.1).

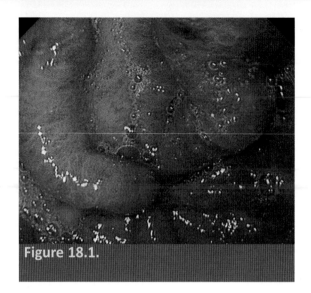

Figure 18.1.

Please describe what you see

This is an endoscopic view of the antrum of the stomach. Classic longitudinal rows of erythematous stripes radiating from the pylorus into the antrum are noted, resembling a watermelon.

What is your diagnosis?

Gastric antral vascular ectasia (GAVE).

Clinical pearls

- GAVE is a rare cause of upper gastrointestinal bleeding.
- It is typically chronic [1] in nature and the patient presents with symptoms of anaemia, although occasionally patients may notice frank melaena or hematochezia.
- The average age of diagnosis is around 70-80 years of age [2], affecting females twice more frequently than males.

The main differential diagnosis is portal hypertensive gastropathy (PHG) (Table 18.1 [3]).

Table 18.1. Features of PHG and GAVE.

Features	PHG	GAVE
Site	Fundus-corpus	Antrum
Endoscopic appearance	Mosaic-like pattern, red point lesions, cherry red spots, black brown spots	Organised red spots in a striped pattern (watermelon stomach)
Histology	Non-specific	Specific
Response to beta-blockers, transjugular intrahepatic portosystemic shunt, portocaval shunts	Present	Absent

Impress your attending

What is the histology of GAVE [4]?
* Vascular ectasia.
* Focal thrombosis.
* Spindle cell proliferation.
* Fibrohyalinosis.

What other diseases is this condition associated with?
* Portal hypertension.
* Chronic renal failure.
* Connective tissue disease (especially systemic sclerosis with positive anti-RNA III polymerase antibodies) [5].

- Bone marrow transplantation.
- Cardiac diseases.

How would you treat this patient?
- Endoscopic treatment:
  - endoscopic coagulation with an argon plasma coagulator (APC) [6];
  - laser photoablation;
  - endoscopic band ligation.
- Antrectomy.

Is APC effective in the treatment of GAVE?
A large series of 100 consecutive patients with gastrointestinal vascular lesions (arteriovenous malformations n = 74, and GAVE n = 26) were treated with APC. APC led to an improvement in median haemoglobin levels, a decreased rate of transfusion per month, with transfusion requirements abolished in 77% of patients [7].

What are the complications of APC?
Complications are rare. The most frequently reported complication is abdominal distension post-procedure. Other rare complications include sepsis, wall emphysema, antral stenosis, perforation and provoking upper gastrointestinal bleeding [8].

References

1. Rosenfeld G, Enns R. Argon photocoagulation in the treatment of gastric antral vascular ectasia and radiation proctitis. *Can J Gastroenterol* 2009; 23(12): 801-4.
2. Nguyen H, Le C, Nguyen H. Gastric antral vascular ectasia (watermelon stomach) - an enigmatic and often-overlooked cause of gastrointestinal bleeding in the elderly. *The Permanente Journal* 2009; 13(4): 46-9.
3. Fuccio L, Mussetto A, Laterza L, *et al.* Diagnosis and management of gastric antral vascular ectasia. *World J Gastrointest Endosc* 2013; 5(1): 6-13.

4. Gilliam JH, Geisinger KR, Wu WC, *et al.* Endoscopic biopsy is diagnostic in gastric antral vascular ectasia. The 'watermelon stomach'. *Dig Dis Sci* 1989; 34: 885-8.
5. Ceribelli A, Cavazzana I, Airo P, Franceschini F. Anti-RNA polymerase III antibodies as a risk marker for early gastric antral vascular ectasia (GAVE) in systemic sclerosis. *J Rheumatol* 2010; 37 (7): 1544.
6. Dulai GS, Jensen DM, Kovacs TO, *et al.* Endoscopic treatment outcomes in watermelon stomach patients with and without portal hypertension. *Endoscopy* 2004; 36: 68-72.
7. Kwan V, Bourke MJ, Williams SJ, *et al.* Argon plasma coagulation in the management of symptomatic gastrointestinal vascular lesions: experience in 100 consecutive patients with long-term follow-up. *Am J Gastroenterol* 2006; 101(1): 58-63.
8. Fuccio L, Mussetto A, Laterza L, *et al.* Diagnosis and management of gastric antral vascular ectasia. *World J Gastrointest Endosc* 2013; 5(1): 6-13.

Case 19

A 54-year-old gentleman with good past health presents with a 2-month history of progressive weight loss, poor appetite and malaise. He has also noted increasing epigastric distension and pain with recurrent vomiting of coffee ground materials. He denies any recent use of non-steroidal anti-inflammatory drugs.

Physical examination

- Afebrile, pulse 70 bpm, BP 125/60mmHg, SaO_2 98-100% on RA.
- Pallor, hydration on the dry side.
- Examination of the hands reveals no clubbing and normal-appearing palmar creases.
- Head and neck examination is unremarkable.
- Cardiovascular: HS dual, no murmur.
- His chest is clear on auscultation.
- Abdominal examination reveals a soft abdomen, with a large mass in the epigastrium, associated with succussion splash.
- No signs of oedema.

Investigations

- CBC:
  - WBC 6.9 x 10^9/L;
  - haemoglobin 6.9g/dL (microcytic hypochromic);
  - platelets 299 x 10^9/L.
- Creatinine 70µmol/L.
- Albumin 33g/L.
- Liver function tests are grossly normal.
- Calcium normal.
- Iron profile: Fe 2µmol/L, TIBC 72µmol/L, Fe saturation <5%.
- pH normal.

What is your clinical diagnosis?

Given the clinical history and examination findings, gastric outlet obstruction (GOO) is suspected. The differential diagnosis would include intestinal obstruction.

What further investigations would you request?

In view of the history of epigastric pain and vomiting, an erect chest X-ray and abdominal X-ray are useful screening tests. The chest X-ray shows no free gas under the diaphragm. The abdominal X-ray is shown below (Figure 19.1).

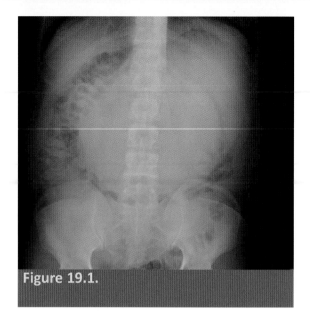

Figure 19.1.

Please describe what you see
There is a large, dilated gastric shadow, likely filled with food contents. This is consistent with a diagnosis of gastric outlet obstruction.

What would be your next step?

The patient should be kept nil per oral, with insertion of a Ryle's tube connected to a bedside bag for gastric decompression, intravenous fluids initiated, and electrolytes corrected.

How would you proceed?

After decompression, an oesophagogastroduodenoscopy (OGD) is arranged. This shows copious amounts of solid food residue in the stomach and a large 3cm x 3cm ulcerative tumour involving the pylorus. This is associated with mucosal oedema and distorted anatomy causing a difficulty for the endoscope to pass through. A guidewire is passed through the narrowing with re-routing of the Ryle's tube performed under fluoroscopic guidance.

What would be your next step of management?

- Tube feeding.
- Proton pump inhibitor.
- Imaging for staging of carcinoma of the stomach, i.e. computed tomography (CT) of the abdomen and pelvis with contrast or positron emission tomography CT (PET-CT).
- Consult the surgery team.

PET-CT images are shown below (Figures 19.2 and 19.3).

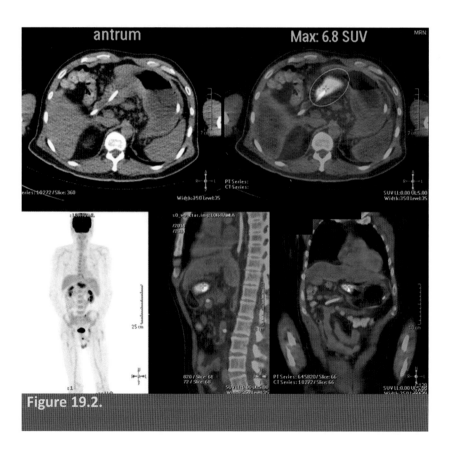

Figure 19.2.

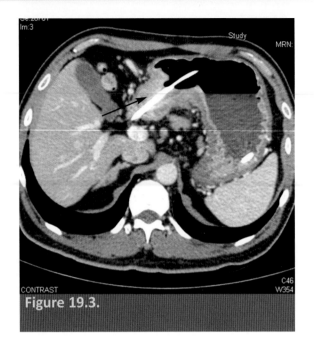

Figure 19.3.

Please describe what you see

There is concentric irregular wall thickening at the gastric antrum measuring 4.2cm long with a maximum standard uptake value (SUVmax) of 6.8. There is no evidence of serosal spread.

There is no other metabolically active metastatic disease noted.

Biopsies show an intestinal type adenocarcinoma of the stomach. In view of localised disease with good functional status, curative resection is arranged.

Clinical pearls

- Gastric outlet obstruction (GOO) is defined as a mechanical impediment to gastric emptying.

- Vomiting is the cardinal symptom. In a patient with epigastric pain, epigastric distension with repeated vomiting, the potential diagnosis of gastric outlet obstruction must be considered. It is important to decompress the stomach prior to endoscopic procedures due to the high risk of aspiration.
- Causes of GOO:
  - benign (39%) [1]:
    - peptic ulcer disease (the most common benign aetiology);
    - gastric polyps;
    - caustic ingestion;
    - pyloric stenosis;
    - congenital duodenal webs;
    - gallstone (Bouveret syndrome);
    - bezoar;
    - pancreatic pseudocysts;
    - Crohn's disease;
  - malignant:
    - peri-pancreatic neoplasms (the most common malignant aetiology);
    - gastric neoplasms;
    - duodenal neoplasms.

Impress your attending

What are the risk factors for stomach cancer [2]?
- *Helicobacter pylori* infection.
- Smoking.
- Preserved foods.
- Obesity.
- Family history of cancer of the stomach.
- Pernicious anaemia.

How would you treat stomach cancer?
Definitive:

- Early disease: endoscopic mucosal resection (EMR) or endoscopic submucosal dissection (ESD).

- Gastrectomy alone, or combined with neoadjuvant chemotherapy or chemoradiation (ECF: epirubicin, cisplatin, 5-fluorouracil [3]) +/- adjuvant chemotherapy or chemoradiation.

Palliative (for unresectable tumours):

- For treatment of the GOO: gastrojejunostomy or self-expandable metallic stents (SEMS).
- Chemotherapy (5-fluorouracil, irinotecan or oxaliplatin-based).
- Targeted therapy, i.e. trastuzumab.

What is trastuzumab?

It is a monoclonal antibody that inhibits the human epidermal growth factor receptor type 2 (HER-2) for tumours that are positive for HER-2.

In a randomised controlled trial published in 2010 [4], trastuzumab in combination with chemotherapy versus chemotherapy alone for HER-2-positive advanced gastric cancers showed a significant difference in median overall survival (13.8 months vs. 11.1 months; hazard ratio 0.74; 95% CI 0.6-0.91; p=0.0046).

What are the newer modalities of treatment on the horizon for advanced gastric cancer?

Immunotherapy is emerging as a new treatment for advanced gastric cancer. A phase Ib trial using pembrolizumab (a humanized monoclonal IgG4 antibody designed to block the interaction between PD-1 and its ligands) showed promising results with 41% of patients experiencing a decrease in tumour burden [5].

References

1. Shone DN, Nikoomanesh P, Smith-Meek MM, Bender JS. Malignancy is the most common cause of gastric outlet obstruction in the era of H2 blockers. *Am J Gastroenterol* 1995; 90: 1769-70.

2. Fuccio L, Eusebi LH, Bazzoli F. Gastric cancer, *Helicobacter pylori* infection and other risk factors. *World J Gastrointest Oncol* 2010; 2(9): 342-7.

3. Cunningham D, Allum WH, Stenning SP, *et al*. Perioperative chemotherapy versus surgery alone for resectable gastroesophageal cancer. *N Engl J Med* 2006; 355: 11-20.

4. Bang YJ, Van Cutsem E, Feyereislova A, *et al*; for the ToGA Trial Investigators. Trastuzumab in combination with chemotherapy versus chemotherapy alone for treatment of HER-2-positive advanced gastric or gastro-oesophageal junction cancer (ToGA): a phase 3, open-label, randomised controlled trial. *Lancet* 2010; 376(9742): 687-97.

5. Muro K, Bang Y, Shankaran V, *et al*. A phase 1b study of pembrolizumab (pembro; MK-3475) in patients with advanced gastric cancer. *Annals Onc* 2014; Suppl 5: v1-v41.

Case 20

History

A 21-year-old lady with a past history of developmental delay and mental retardation is admitted for coffee ground vomiting. She has had multiple readmissions for a similar problem. She has normal bowel motions and flatus. There is no other significant past medical history.

Physical examination

- Afebrile, pulse 72 bpm, BP 115/80mmHg, SaO_2 98-100% on RA.
- Hydration is satisfactory.
- Examination of the hands reveals no clubbing and normal-appearing palmar creases.
- Head and neck examination is unremarkable.
- Cardiovascular: HS dual, no murmur.
- Her chest is clear on auscultation.
- Abdominal examination reveals a distended abdomen, but no frank peritoneal signs could be elicited. Bowel sounds are sluggish.
- No signs of oedema.

Investigations

- CBC:
  - WBC 9.9×10^9/L;
  - haemoglobin 13.1g/dL;
  - platelets 289×10^9/L.
- Electrolytes are grossly normal.
- Bone profile is normal.
- Amylase 113 IU/L.
- pH 7.43.
- BE -2.
- sTSH 3.78mIU/L.

An abdominal X-ray is also performed (Figure 20.1).

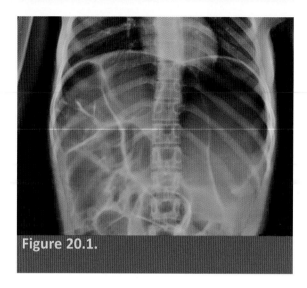

Figure 20.1.

Please describe what you see
There are markedly dilated large bowel loops.

What is your differential diagnosis?

Mechanical:

- Large bowel intestinal obstruction.
- Colonic volvulus.

Non-mechanical:

- Acute:
  - acute intestinal pseudo-obstruction (Ogilvie's syndrome);
  - toxic megacolon (usually in ulcerative colitis, pseudomembranous colitis).
- Chronic intestinal pseudo-obstruction (CIPO).

What further investigations may be helpful?

- Computed tomography of the abdomen (which is negative in this case for any transition point or obstructive lesion).

- Endoscopy.
- Functional assessments (i.e. transit studies, manometry).
- Barium or water-soluble contrast studies (i.e. small bowel follow-through, barium enema).
- Full-thickness biopsies.

What is the likely diagnosis?

In view of the recurrent nature with no mechanical cause identified, the most likely diagnosis is chronic intestinal pseudo-obstruction.

Clinical pearls

- Chronic intestinal pseudo-obstruction (CIPO) is a rare condition with no specific biomarkers. A detailed history, physical examination, laboratory tests and radiological investigations are needed to exclude other potentially reversible diagnoses.
- CIPO is characterised by a high morbidity (significant pain symptoms, malnutrition) and mortality (i.e. total parenteral nutrition complications, surgical complications, sepsis from gastrointestinal origin) [1]. Long-term outcomes are usually poor despite treatment.
- Treatment of CIPO focuses mainly on:
  - nutritional support +/- parenteral nutrition;
  - pharmacological: prokinetic agents such as erythromycin, metoclopramide, octreotide or neostigmine may be useful in controlling symptoms;
  - surgical, i.e. gastrostomy or enterostomy can be considered in rare cases with localised involvement of the gastrointestinal tract;
  - intestinal transplantation (only available in highly specialised centres) [2].

Impress your attending

What is the postulated pathogenesis in chronic intestinal pseudo-obstruction?

It is thought to arise from abnormalities in gut peristalsis, either from dysfunction of smooth muscles of the gut (myopathy), interstitial cells of Cajal (mesenchymopathy) or the nervous system (neuropathy).

How would you classify the causes of CIPO (Table 20.1)?

Table 20.1. Classification of the causes of CIPO.

Primary	Secondary
Myopathy	Infective (Chagas disease)
Mesenchymopathy (interstitial cells of Cajal)	Collagen vascular disease (systemic sclerosis, systemic lupus erythematosus, mixed connective
Neuropathy (Hirschsprung's)	tissue disorder, etc.)
	Endocrine disorders (diabetes mellitus, hypothyroidism, hypoparathyroidism)
	Medication-associated (tricyclic antidepressants, anticholinergics)
	Paraneoplastic (small cell lung carcinoma, carcinoids, lymphoma)
	Infiltrative diseases (lymphoma, amyloidosis)
	Neurological disorders (Parkinson's, stroke, encephalitis, basal ganglia calcification)

What is Hirschsprung's disease?

It is a congenital malformation characterised by the absence of parasympathetic intrinsic ganglion cells in the submucosal and myenteric plexuses [3].

References

1. Antonucci A, Fronzoni L, Cogliandro L, *et al*. Chronic intestinal pseudo-obstruction. *World J Gastroenterol* 2008; 14(19): 2953-61.
2. Stanghellini V, Cogliandro R, Giorgio R, *et al*. Natural history of chronic idiopathic intestinal pseudo-obstruction in adults: a single center study. *Clin Gastro Hep* 2005; 3: 449-58.
3. Whitehouse F, Kernohan J. Myenteric plexuses in congenital megacolon; study of 11 cases. *Arch Intern Med* 1948; 82: 75.

Case 21

An 80-year-old gentleman with a past history of diabetes, hypertension, hyperlipidaemia and chronic kidney disease is admitted with symptoms of epigastric pain. On further enquiry, he also reveals a history of prophylactic colectomy for familial adenomatous polyposis.

Physical examination

- Afebrile, pulse 64 bpm, BP 135/60mmHg, SaO_2 98-100% on RA.
- Hydration is good.
- Examination of the hands reveals no clubbing and normal-appearing palmar creases.
- Head and neck examination is unremarkable.
- Cardiovascular: HS dual, no murmur.
- His chest is clear on auscultation.
- Abdominal examination reveals a soft abdomen, with a midline laparotomy scar noted.
- No signs of oedema.

Investigations

- CBC:
  - WBC 7.2 x 10^9/L;
  - haemoglobin 10.9g/dL;
  - platelets 191 x 10^9/L.
- Creatinine 123µmol/L.
- Liver function tests are normal.
- Clotting profile is normal.

What would you do next?

An oesophagogastroduodenoscopy (OGD) should be performed (Figures 21.1 and 21.2).

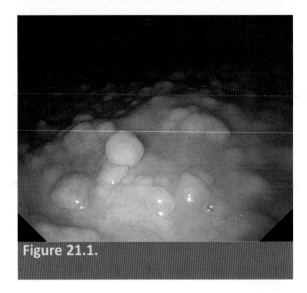

Figure 21.1.

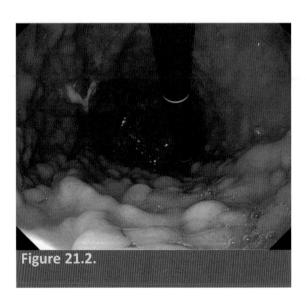

Figure 21.2.

Please describe what you see

There are multiple, small 2-4mm, sessile polyps with a smooth surface throughout the entire stomach, mainly concentrated at the fundus and body upon retroflexion of the endoscope.

What is your differential diagnosis?

- Fundic gland polyp.
- Hyperplastic polyp.
- Hamartomatous polyp.
- Adenomatous polyp.

How would you proceed?

- Biopsy the lesions.
- Drug history — any long-term use of proton pump inhibitors.

The biopsy results show some dilated fundic glands lined by an attenuated layer of chief and parietal cells with no features of dysplasia or malignancy, in keeping with the diagnosis of fundic gland polyps.

Clinical pearls

- Fundic gland polyps (FGP) are one of the most commonly found polyps in the stomach. They are reported to be found in 0.8-23% of endoscopies [1].
- They are observed in three clinical contexts:
  - sporadic;
  - proton pump inhibitor use [2];
  - syndromic:
    - familial adenomatous polyposis (FAP) or attenuated FAP;
    - Zollinger-Ellison syndrome.

- Atypical features of FGPs include:
  - young age <40 years;
  - sites other than the fundus and body;
  - size >1cm;
  - eroded or ulcerated surface;
  - numerous, i.e. n ≥20;
  - associated with duodenal adenoma or abnormal papilla.

If such features are present, dysplasia and/or neoplasia needs to be considered. Colonoscopy to exclude FAP or attenuated FAP is warranted.

Impress your attending

Which gene is affected in FAP?
The disease is caused by a germline mutation in the adenomatous polyposis coli (APC) gene on chromosome 5q21 [3].

Inheritance is autosomal dominant with high penetrance. De novo mutations arise in around 20% of cases.

How is classic FAP diagnosed?
- Clinical criteria: an individual having more than 100 adenomatous colonic polyps diagnosed before the age of 40.
- Genetic testing: APC gene on chromosome 5.

Which types of multiple colorectal adenoma syndromes do you know of?

Classic FAP (>100 adenomas)
Many patients have hundreds, often thousands of adenomatous polyps by the age of 40. The lifetime risk of colorectal carcinoma (CRC) in classic FAP approaches 100% [4]. The mean age of CRC diagnosis in untreated individuals is 39 years. Therefore, colectomy is recommended to reduce the risk of CRC (Figure 21.3).

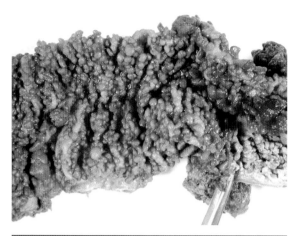

Figure 21.3.

Attenuated FAP

This condition is characterised by the presence of fewer than 100 polyps, a more proximal colonic distribution of polyps, and a later development of CRC (15 years later than patients with classic FAP). The cumulative risk of CRC by the age of 80 years is around 69% [5].

MYH-associated polyposis

This is an autosomal recessive type of polyposis, involving the human MutY homologue (MYH) gene, which is located on chromosome 1p [6].

What are the clinical presentations of classic FAP [7]?

- Colon:
  - adenomatous polyps and CRC (metastatic CRC is the leading cause of death).
- Upper gastrointestinal tract:
  - adenomatous polyps (advanced duodenal adenomas may lead to small bowel cancer, a third leading cause of death);
  - fundic gland polyps/fundic gland polyposis.
- Desmoid tumours, usually intra-abdominal (a second leading cause of death).

- Thyroid cancer.
- Hepatoblastoma in children.
- Congenital hypertrophy of retinal pigmented epithelium (usually asymptomatic with no malignant potential. It is specific for FAP and has been associated with increased severity).

Which eponymous syndromes are related with FAP?

- Gardner syndrome:
  - association of polyposis, with soft tissue tumours such as epidermoid cysts, fibromas, lipomas, desmoids tumours and bone abnormalities such as osteomas.
- Turcot syndrome:
  - association of polyposis, with a primary central nervous system tumour.

What are the latest recommendations for colorectal cancer (CRC) screening for patients with FAP [8]?

According to the latest American College of Gastroenterology (ACG) guidelines for CRC screening published in 2009:

- Patients with classic FAP (>100 adenomas) should be advised to seek genetic counselling and, if appropriate, genetic testing. If APC mutation testing is negative, MYH mutation testing is recommended.
- Patients with known FAP or who are at risk of FAP based on family history (and genetic testing has not been performed) should undergo annual flexible sigmoidoscopy or colonoscopy, as appropriate (previous guidelines recommended screening from age 10-12 years onwards [9]), until colectomy is deemed by the physician and patient as the best treatment.
- Patients with a retained rectum after a subtotal colectomy should undergo flexible sigmoidoscopy every 6-12 months.
- Upper endoscopic surveillance has also been recommended for individuals with FAP or MYH-associated polyposis.

References

1. Islam RS, Patel NC, Lam-Himlin D, Nguyen CC. Gastric polyps: a review of clinical, endoscopic, and histopathologic features and management decisions. *Gastroenterol Hepatol (NY)* 2013; 9(10): 640-51.
2. Choudhry U, Boyce HW, Coppola D. Proton pump inhibitor-associated gastric polyps: a retrospective analysis of their frequency, and endoscopic, histologic, and ultrastructural characteristics. *Am J Clin Pathol* 1998; 110: 615-21.
3. Bodmer WF, Bailey CJ, Bodmer J, *et al.* Localization of the gene for familial adenomatous polyposis on chromosome 5. *Nature* 1987; 328: 614-6.
4. Bisgaard ML, Fenger K, Bulow S, *et al.* Familial adenomatous polyposis (FAP): frequency, penetrance, and mutation rate. *Hum Mutat* 1994; 3: 121-5.
5. Burt RW, Leppert MF, Slattery ML, *et al.* Genetic testing and phenotype in a large kindred with attenuated familial adenomatous polyposis. *Gastroenterology* 2004; 127: 444-51.
6. Sampson JR, Dolwani S, Jones S, *et al.* Autosomal recessive colorectal adenomatous polyposis due to inherited mutations of MYH. *Lancet* 2003; 362: 39-41.
7. Galiatsatos P, Foulkes WD. Familial adenomatous polyposis. *Am J Gastroenterol* 2006; 101(2): 385-98.
8. Rex DK, Johnson DA, Anderson JC, *et al*; for the American College of Gastroenterology. American College of Gastroenterology guidelines for colorectal cancer screening. *Am J Gastroenterol* 2009; 104(3): 739-50.
9. Winawer S, Fletcher R, Rex D, *et al.* U.S. Multisociety Task Force on Colorectal Cancer. Colorectal cancer screening and surveillance: Clinical guidelines and rationale - update based on new evidence. *Gastroenterology* 2003; 124: 544-60.

Case 22

A 88-year-old gentleman from a nursing home is brought to the accident and emergency department after ingestion of a foreign body. The caregiver suspects he had swallowed a five dollar coin (Figure 22.1). He subsequently develops chest pain and epigastric discomfort hours after ingestion. He has a past history of hypertension, diabetes mellitus and dementia.

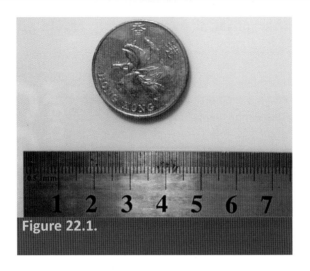

Figure 22.1.

Physical examination

- Afebrile, pulse 94 bpm, BP 160/80mmHg, SaO_2 98% on RA.
- Hydration is satisfactory.
- Examination of the hands reveals no clubbing and normal-appearing palmar creases.
- Head and neck examination is unremarkable.
- Cardiovascular: HS dual, no murmur.
- His chest is clear on auscultation, with no stridor. He is not in respiratory distress.
- Abdominal examination reveals a soft abdomen, with no tenderness/guarding/rebound tenderness. Bowel sounds are normal.
- No signs of oedema.

Investigations

- CBC:
  - WBC 7.9 x 10^9/L;
  - haemoglobin 13g/dL;
  - platelets 226 x 10^9/L.
- Liver function tests are normal.
- CRP normal.
- Clotting profile is normal.

What other physical examinations would you like to perform?

A complete neck exam looking for erythema, tenderness, swelling or crepitus should be performed. If crepitus is present it would be suggestive of subcutaneous emphysema and raises the suspicion of a perforated viscus.

What further investigations would you request?

Radiographs would be useful for localisation and screening for complications, such as free gas under the diaphragm or mediastinal gas.

A lateral radiograph of the neck together with a chest X-ray are performed (Figure 22.2).

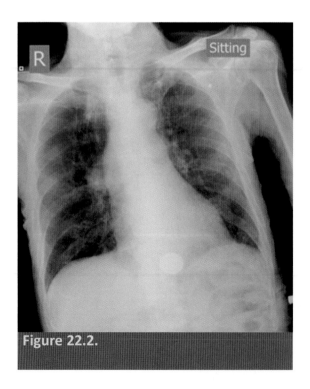

Figure 22.2.

Please describe what you see

This is an anterior-posterior (AP) chest radiograph showing a radio-opaque, circular, well-circumscribed lesion at the lower mediastinum above the right hemi-diaphragm. It is likely to correspond with the level of the distant oesophagus.

A diagnosis of foreign body ingestion (coin) is made.

How would you manage this gentleman?

In view of worsening symptoms, it is decided that an oesophagogastro-duodenoscopy (OGD) with removal of the foreign body is important for symptomatic relief.

The following image is an endoscopic view (Figure 22.3).

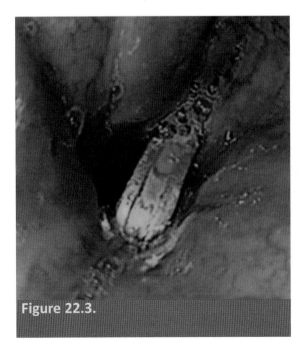

Figure 22.3.

Please describe what you see

The endoscopic view shows an impacted coin at the distal oesophagogastric junction (OGJ). This is gently pushed into the stomach and subsequently removed by a retrieval net.

The remainder of the upper digestive tract is examined again with no frank pathology noted.

Clinical pearls

- Foreign body ingestion is commonly found in paediatric populations [1], and adults who have alcoholic intoxication, psychiatric disorders or mental impairment [2].
- Initial assessment must include an assessment of the airway, with consideration of endotracheal intubation for airway protection if appropriate, i.e. unable to manage secretions and at high aspiration risk. A physical exam specifically to look for oesophageal perforation, peritoneal signs, and signs of intestinal obstruction are also warranted.
- Sites where there is narrowing or angulation may lead to impaction, perforation or obstruction. These could include normal sites such as the distal OGJ, pylorus and terminal ileum [3]. Sites of previous gastrointestinal tract surgery or congenital gut malformation are also at high risk [4].
- Retrieval devices such as alligator forceps, polypectomy snares, Dormia® baskets, retrieval nets, magnet probes, etc., have all been used to remove foreign bodies. Overtubes are sometimes deployed to protect the airway, facilitate passage of the endoscope during removal of the foreign body, and to protect the oesophageal mucosa from laceration during retrieval of sharp objects [5].

Impress your attending

Are there any specific foreign bodies where endoscopic removal should not be attempted, and why?
Narcotic/drug-containing packets in drug traffickers.

This is due to the potentially fatal consequences if there is rupture or leakage of the contents within such packages. Direct surgical intervention is indicated if there is impaction of the packets or signs and symptoms of intestinal obstruction occur [6].

What factors would you take into account when considering timing of endoscopy?

With reference to the American Society for Gastrointestinal Endoscopy (ASGE) guidelines, the management of ingested foreign bodies and food impactions is shown below (Figure 22.4 [7]).

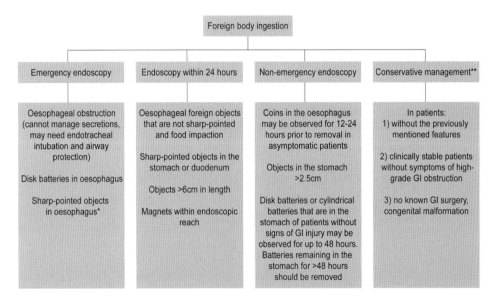

* Ingestion of sharp pointed objects in the oesophagus is a medical emergency. Even if the object has passed into the stomach the risk of complications are still approximately 35% [8].
** Once a foreign body enters the stomach, most objects pass in 4 to 6 days [9]. Regular diet can be continued and observation of stools for evidence of passing of the foreign body. Weekly radiographs are recommended.

Figure 22.4. American Society for Gastrointestinal Endoscopy (ASGE) guidelines on the management of ingested foreign bodies and food impaction.

References

1. Hachimi-Idrissi S, Come L, Vandenpias Y. Management of ingested foreign bodies in childhood: our experience and review of the literature. *Eur J Emerg Med* 1998; 5: 319-23.
2. Webb WA. Management of foreign bodies of the upper gastrointestinal tract: update. *Gastrointest Endosc* 1995; 41: 39-51.
3. Goh BK, Chow PK, Quah HM, *et al*. Perforation of the gastrointestinal tract secondary to ingestion of foreign bodies. *World J Surg* 2006; 30(3): 372-7.
4. Ginsberg GG. Management of ingested foreign objects and food bolus impactions. *Gastrointest Endosc* 1995; 41: 33-8.
5. ASGE Technology Committee, Tierney WM, Adler DC, Conway JD, *et al*. Overtube use in gastrointestinal endoscopy. *Gastrointest Endosc* 2009; 70: 828-34.
6. Lancashire MJR, Legg PK, Lowe M, *et al*. Surgical aspects of international drug smuggling. *BMJ* 1988; 296: 1035-7.
7. ASGE Standards of Practice Committee, Ikenberry SO, Jue TL, Anderson MA, *et al*. Management of ingested foreign bodies and food impactions. *Gastrointest Endosc* 2011; 73(6): 1085-91.
8. Carp L. Foreign bodies in the intestine. *Ann Surg* 1927; 85: 575-91.
9. Bendig DW, Machel GO. Management of smooth-blunt gastric foreign bodies in asymptomatic patients. *Clin Pediatr* 1990; 29: 642-5.

Case 23

A 63-year-old Chinese gentleman with a past history of aortic stenosis and cholangitis with a previous cholecystectomy presents with right upper quadrant pain radiating to the back and tea-coloured urine. He also reports chills and rigors.

Physical examination

- Temperature 38°C, pulse 70 bpm, BP 129/64mmHg, SaO_2 98-100% on RA.
- Hydration is satisfactory.
- Examination of the hands reveals no clubbing and normal-appearing palmar creases.
- Head and neck examination is unremarkable.
- Cardiovascular: HS dual, no murmur.
- His chest is clear on auscultation.
- Abdominal examination reveals a soft abdomen, with right upper quadrant tenderness. Murphy's sign is negative.
- No signs of oedema.

Investigations

- CBC:
  - WBC 11.7 x 10^9/L;
  - haemoglobin 13.3g/dL;
  - platelets 294 x 10^9/L.
- Bilirubin 35µmol/L.
- ALP 123 IU/L.
- ALT 221 IU/L.
- Clotting profile is normal.
- Amylase 98 IU/L.
- Blood gases: no acidosis.
- A screening chest X-ray and abdominal X-ray are also done which are normal.

What is your working diagnosis?

In view of the right upper quadrant pain, tea-coloured urine, fever and deranged liver function tests, biliary obstruction needs to be excluded.

How would you proceed?

Imaging including ultrasonography of the hepatobiliary and pancreatic system (USG HBP) or computed tomography with contrast of the abdomen are initial investigations for biliary obstruction.

A USG HBP is done, showing a 1.8cm dilated common bile duct and dilated intrahepatic ducts but the distal common bile duct is obscured.

What would you do next?

- Fluid resuscitation.
- Empirical broad-spectrum antibiotics.
- Endoscopic retrograde cholangiopancreatography (ERCP) for biliary drainage.

A cholangiogram is shown below (Figure 23.1).

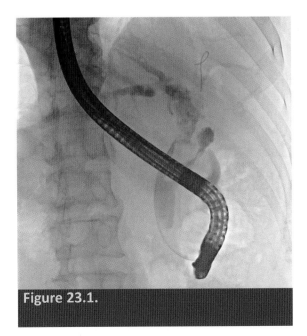

Figure 23.1.

Please describe what you see

The fluoroscopic image shows the common bile duct 2cm in diameter with a large elongated stone (2.5cm x 2cm) in the mid common bile duct. The intrahepatic ducts also show dilatation.

What would be your diagnosis?

In view of repeated attacks of cholangitis despite having a cholecystectomy, together with the cholangiogram findings, recurrent pyogenic cholangitis is suspected.

Clinical pearls

- Recurrent pyogenic cholangitis (RPC), also known as oriental cholangiohepatitis or Hong Kong disease, is characterised by de novo intrabiliary pigment stone formation causing recurrent bouts of cholangitis, which results in stricturing of the biliary tree and biliary obstruction. Long-term complications include secondary biliary cirrhosis and cholangiocarcinoma.
- The left hepatic duct (left lateral segmental duct) is usually affected early during the course of the disease. This may be due to the more acute angle of these ducts predisposing to stasis and strictures [1]. It is a differential diagnosis of recurrent attacks of cholangitis especially in individuals of Southeast Asian descent [2]. It is reported that stones recur in >30% of patients [3].
- The pathogenesis has yet to be fully elucidated, but it is postulated to be related to:
  - biliary helminths — inflammation and ductal injury secondary to parasitic infections. Commonly implicated species include *Clonorchis sinensis* [4] and *Ascaris lumbricoides*;
  - transient portal bacteraemia — inflammation from secondary bacterial infections may lead to recurrent attacks of cholangitis. Some enteric bacteria with beta-glucuronidase activity may cause deconjugation of bilirubin glucuronide, leading to the precipitation of bilirubin pigment stones inside the biliary ducts;
  - malnutrition.

- A low protein diet may lead to decreased levels of endogenously produced inhibitors of beta-glucuronidase activity, leading to increased suspectibility of bilirubin pigment stone formation.

Impress your attending

What are the typical cholangiographic findings [5]?
Typical cholangiographic findings include:

- Intrahepatic and extrahepatic duct dilatation.
- Straightening of intrahepatic ducts with an increase in angle or even right-angled branching patterns.
- Arrowhead sign: decreased arborisation and acute tapering of the peripheral ducts.
- Missing duct sign.

How would you manage these patients in the long term?
- Removal of stones endoscopically followed by regular surveillance.
- Surgical resection of the affected liver segment.

References

1. Cosenza CA, Durazo F, Stain SC, *et al.* Current management of recurrent pyogenic cholangitis. *Am Surg* 1999; 65: 939.
2. Ong GB. A study of recurrent pyogenic cholangitis. *Arch Surg* 1962; 84: 199.
3. Cheng YF, Lee TY, Sheen-Chen SM, *et al.* Treatment of complicated hepatolithiasis with intrahepatic biliary stricture by ductal dilatation and stenting: long-term results. *World J Surg* 2000; 24: 712.
4. Lim JH. Radiologic findings of clonorchiasis. *AJR Am J Roentgenol* 1990; 155: 1001.
5. Khuroo MS, Dar MY, Yattoo GN, *et al.* Serial cholangiographic appearances in recurrent pyogenic cholangitis. *Gastrointest Endosc* 1993; 39: 674.

Case 24

History

A 64-year-old gentleman presents with increasing right upper abdominal swelling and discomfort. He denies any constitutional symptoms, and there are no symptoms of fever, chills or rigors. He has a history of hypertension.

Physical examination

- Afebrile, pulse 98 bpm, BP 142/89mmHg, SaO$_2$ 98-100% on RA.
- Tired-looking, hydration on the dry side.
- Examination of the hands reveals no clubbing and normal-appearing palmar creases.
- Head and neck examination is unremarkable.
- Cardiovascular: HS dual, no murmur.
- His chest is clear on auscultation.
- Abdominal examination reveals a soft abdomen, mild right upper quadrant tenderness, gross hepatomegaly with a lobulated surface.
- No stigmata of chronic liver disease.
- No signs of oedema.

Investigations

- CBC is normal.
- Liver and renal function tests are normal.
- CRP normal.
- HBsAg, anti-HCV negative.

What is your differential diagnosis?

- Neoplasm:
    - primary, i.e. hepatocellular carcinoma, cholangiocarcinoma;
    - secondary metastases.
- Liver abscess.
- Liver cysts:
    - simple cysts;
    - congenital, i.e. polycystic kidney and liver disease or polycystic liver disease.

What would you do next?

Structural imaging of the abdomen would be helpful in delineating the various causes of hepatomegaly, i.e. ultrasonography or a computed tomography (CT) scan with contrast of the abdomen.

The following CT images are obtained (Figures 24.1 and 24.2).

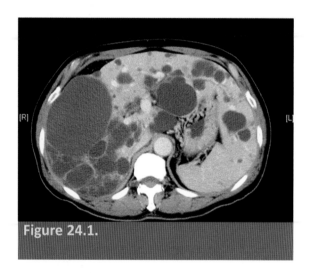

Figure 24.1.

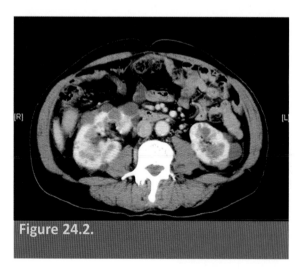

Figure 24.2.

Please describe what you see

There are multiple liver cysts in both hepatic lobes with gross hepatomegaly. There is no abnormal cyst wall thickening or hyperdense content which suggests recent infection or haemorrhage. The biliary tree is not dilated.

There are also multiple cysts of variable size in both kidneys. There is no abnormal cyst wall thickening or enhancing solid components.

What is the likely diagnosis?

Autosomal dominant polycystic kidney disease with liver involvement.

Clinical pearls

- Polycystic liver disease (PCLD) can present as an extrarenal manifestation in autosomal dominant polycystic kidney disease.
- The majority of patients with polycystic liver disease are asymptomatic [1], but they can also present with a myriad of symptoms:
  - mechanical symptoms, i.e. abdominal discomfort, pain, distension, postprandial fullness, shortness of breath;
  - acute pain may be due to cyst rupture, haemorrhage or infection;
  - cysts may also cause compression of the biliary tree and hepatic venous outflow, leading to obstructive jaundice or portal hypertension.
- If there is kidney involvement, other presentations such as haematuria, urinary tract infection and infected renal cysts, renal cyst haemorrhage, and progressive renal failure may also be present.

Impress your attending

What is the definition of polycystic liver disease?
It is arbituarily defined as a liver that contains >20 cysts [2].

What are the genetic diseases and corresponding genes associated with this condition?

Isolated polycystic liver disease (PCLD) is associated with mutations in the PRKCSH and SEC63 genes.

Extrarenal manifestations of autosomal dominant polycystic kidney disease (ADPKD) are associated with mutations in the PKD1 and PKD2 genes.

What are the risk factors for the growth of liver cysts [3, 4]?
- Female sex.
- Multiparity.
- Exogenous oestrogen use.

What are the treatment strategies that can be implemented for symptomatic PCLD [5]?

Treatment of liver cysts is aimed at reducing the volume of the diseased liver with the aim of improving symptoms [6]:

- Aspiration sclerotherapy.
- Surgical cyst deroofing.
- Liver transplantation.

Do you know of any pharmacological options that may be useful in this condition [7]?

Using a somatostatin analogue, lanreotide, Chrispijn *et al* were able to demonstrate a reduction in liver volume by 4% (IQR -6% to -1%) after 12 months of treatment. However, stopping the treatment leads to a recurrence of polycystic liver growth.

References

1. Qian Q, Li A, King BF, *et al*. Clinical profile of autosomal dominant polycystic liver disease. *Hepatology* 2003; 37(1): 164-71.
2. Drenth JP, Chrispijn M, Nagorney DM, *et al*. Medical and surgical treatment options for polycystic liver disease. *Hepatology* 2010; 52: 2223-30.

3. Sherstha R, McKinley C, Russ P, *et al.* Postmenopausal estrogen therapy selectively stimulates hepatic enlargement in women with autosomal dominant polycystic kidney disease. *Hepatology* 1997; 26: 1282-6.

4. Chapman AB. Cystic disease in women: clinical characteristics and medical management. *Adv Ren Replace Ther* 2003; 10: 24-30.

5. Cnossen WR, Drenth JP. Polycystic liver disease: an overview of pathogenesis, clinical manifestations and management. *Orphanet J Rare Dis* 2014; 9: 69.

6. van Keimpema L, Hockerstedt K. Treatment of polycystic liver disease. *Br J Surg* 2009; 96: 1379-80.

7. Chrispijn M, Nevens F, Gevers TJ, *et al.* The long-term outcome of patients with polycystic liver disease treated with lanreotide. *Aliment Pharmacol Ther* 2012; 35(2): 266-74.

Case 25

A 60-year-old lady with a past history of diabetes mellitus and chronic hepatitis B presents with progressive weight loss of 2kg over 3 months associated with non-specific abdominal discomfort. She is a non-drinker.

Physical examination

- Afebrile, pulse 80 bpm, BP 120/80mmHg, SaO_2 98-100% on RA.
- Hydration is satisfactory.
- Examination of the hands reveals no clubbing and normal-appearing palmar creases.
- Head and neck examination is unremarkable.
- Cardiovascular: HS dual, no murmur.
- Her chest is clear on auscultation.
- Abdominal examination reveals a soft, non-tender abdomen, with no peritoneal signs.
- No signs of oedema.

Investigations

- CBC:
  - WBC 6.2 x 10^9/L;
  - haemoglobin 12.3g/dL;
  - platelets 262 x 10^9/L.

A computed tomography scan is performed (Figure 25.1).

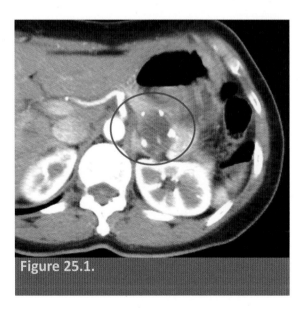

Figure 25.1.

Please describe what you see

A cystic lesion is noted at the pancreatic tail (circle). There are irregular peripheral calcifications noted.

What is your differential diagnosis?

- Mucinous cystic neoplasm (MCN).
- Serous cystic neoplasm (SCN).
- Intraductal papillary mucinous neoplasm (IPMN).

How would you proceed?

As the diagnosis is not clear at this juncture, further investigation with endoscopic ultrasound (EUS) (Figure 25.2) would be helpful in differentiating the various types of pancreatic cystic neoplasms. This could be achieved by the ultrasonographic appearance, together with EUS-guided fine-needle aspiration for cytology (FNAC) and cyst fluid analysis.

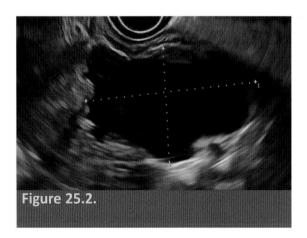

Figure 25.2.

Please describe what you see

There is a 4.2cm x 2.8cm well defined cystic lesion with a few septations at the pancreatic tail. Fine-needle aspiration is performed which reveals that the fluid is compatible with cystic fluid, but no epithelial lining or malignant cells could be found.

Does this narrow the differential?

Thin septations are usually found in mucinous cystic neoplasms.

What would you do next?

In view of the suspected mucinous cystic neoplasm, the large size of the lesion, accompanied by constitutional symptoms of weight loss, in a woman with a relatively good functional status, she is referred to the surgical department for resection.

What is the final pathological diagnosis?

The following histological images are shown in Figures 25.3 and 25.4.

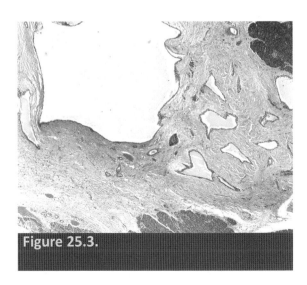

Figure 25.3.

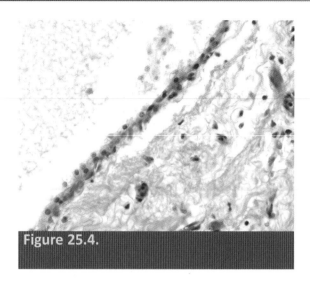

Figure 25.4.

Please describe what you see
The low-power view (Figure 25.3) shows a multiloculated macrocystic and microcystic pancreatic lesion. The high-power view (Figure 25.4) shows benign cuboidal cells with clear or eosinophilic cytoplasm.

What is your final diagnosis?

Serous cystadenoma.

Clinical pearls

- Pancreatic cystic lesions are diagnosed more frequently due to the increasing use and resolution of cross-sectional imaging.
- Important diagnostic modalities include cross-sectional imaging (computed tomography or magnetic resonance imaging) and endoscopic ultrasound +/- image-guided FNAC and cyst fluid analysis [1].
- The typical features of a serous cystadenoma on a CT scan are a honeycomb appearance (due to multiple microcystic tumours) and sunburst calcifications (central stellate scar) for the microcystic variant (cysts <5mm). The macrocystic variant (cysts >5mm) is less common.
- For a mucinous cystic neoplasm, septations and eggshell calcification are characteristic.

- Intraductal papillary mucinous neoplasms (IPMN) can be classified as branch duct and main duct IPMNs. Branch duct IPMNs are characterised by dilated side branches with communication with the main pancreatic duct. For main duct IPMNs, endoscopic examination may reveal a fish-mouth appearance of the ampulla with mucin extrusion and a dilated tortuous main pancreatic duct with filling defects (which may represent mural nodules, papillary tumours or mucin globules).

Impress your attending

How would you interpret cyst fluid analysis in pancreatic cystic lesions (Table 25.1 [2])?

Table 25.1. Interpretation of investigations for pancreatic cyst fluid.

	Pseudocyst	Serous cyst-adenoma	MCN-benign	MCN-malignant	IPMN
Viscosity	Low	Low	High	High	High
Amylase	High	Low	Low	Low	High
CEA	Low	Low	High	High	High
CA 72-4	Low	Low	Intermediate	High	Intermediate to high
Cytology	Histiocytes	Cuboid cells with glycogen-rich cytoplasm	Columnar mucinous epithelial cells with variable atypia	Adenocarcinoma cells	Columnar mucinous epithelial cells with variable atypia

CEA: carcinoembryonic antigen; CA: cancer antigen; IPMN: intraductal papillary mucinous neoplasm; MCN: mucinous cystic neoplasm.

When is resection indicated for pancreatic cystic lesions?

For MCN and IPMN, the updated Fukuoka Consensus Guidelines by Tanaka *et al*, updated in 2012 [3], provide a good framework to guide management, but ultimately the decision for surgery or conservative management requires an individualised approach, taking into consideration premorbid status, life expectancy and the malignant potential of the lesion [1].

Worrisome features — proceed with EUS for risk stratification:

- Cyst size ≥3cm.
- Main pancreatic duct (MPD) 5-9mm.
- Thickened or enhancing cyst wall.
- Abrupt change in calibre of the MPD with distal pancreatic atrophy.
- Suspected non-enhancing mural nodule.
- Lymphadenopathy.
- Pancreatitis.
- If EUS detects a definite mural nodule, MPD involvement or positive cytology, surgery should be considered.

High-risk stigmata — surgery should be considered:

- Obstructive jaundice in a patient with a cystic lesion in the pancreatic head.
- MPD >10mm.
- Enhancing solid component/mural nodule.

References

1. Tang RS, Savides TJ. Pancreatic cystic lesions. *Gastrointestinal Endoscopy in the Cancer Patient*, 1st ed. Oxford, UK: Blackwell Publishing Ltd: 147-60.
2. *Sleisenger & Fordtran's Gastrointestinal and Liver Disease*, 9th ed. Philadelphia, USA: Saunders, 2010.
3. Tanaka M, Fernández-del Castillo C, Adsay V, *et al*; International Association of Pancreatology. International consensus guidelines 2012 for the management of IPMN and MCN of the pancreas. *Pancreatology* 2012; 12(3): 183-97.

Case 26

History

A 64-year-old gentleman who is an ex-heavy smoker and chronic drinker presents with painless progressive dysphagia over the past few months. There is also weight loss and a decrease in appetite. He denies any symptoms of gastrointestinal bleeding.

Physical examination

- Afebrile, pulse 80 bpm, BP 120/80mmHg, SaO_2 98-100% on RA.
- Hydration is satisfactory.
- Examination of the hands reveals no clubbing and normal-appearing palmar creases.
- Head and neck examination is unremarkable.
- Cardiovascular: HS dual, no murmur.
- His chest is clear on auscultation.
- Abdominal examination reveals a soft, non-tender abdomen, with no peritoneal signs.
- No signs of oedema.

Investigations

- CBC:
  - WBC 8.2 x 10^9/L;
  - haemoglobin 12.5g/dL;
  - platelets 294 x 10^9/L.
- Urea 4.6mmol/L.
- Liver function tests are normal.
- Renal function tests are grossly unremarkable.
- Clotting profile is normal.

What further investigation would you perform?

In view of the symptoms of dysphagia associated with mild anaemia, an oesophagogastroduodenoscopy (OGD) is warranted (Figure 26.1).

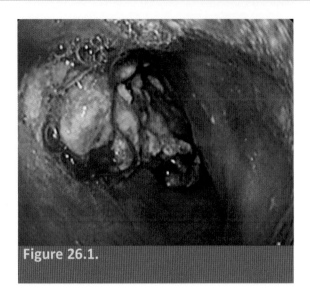

Figure 26.1.

Please describe what you see

A circumferential ulcerative obstructing tumour growth is noted in the mid-oesophagus. The 9.8mm endoscope could not pass; therefore, a 5mm nasoendoscope is used, which is able to negotiate past the obstructing tumour, revealing that the tumour spans ~10cm (from 24cm to 34cm from the incisors). Multiple biopsies are taken.

What would you do next?

In view of the obstructing tumour with symptoms of dysphagia, an endoscopy-guided feeding tube is inserted to provide nutrition.

The following is a histological photo (Figure 26.2).

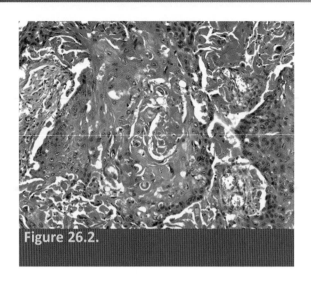

Figure 26.2.

Please describe what you see

The above image shows fragments of squamous carcinoma cells arranged in sheets and nests with keratinisation.

How would you proceed?

Staging would be required for consideration of further management options.

Positron electron tomography-computed tomography scans are arranged (Figures 26.3 and 26.4).

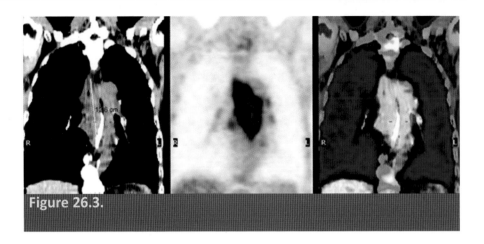

Figure 26.3.

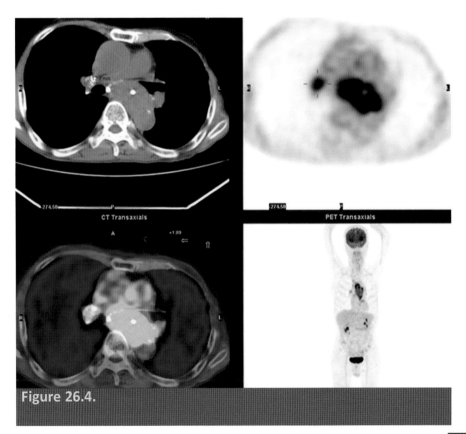

Figure 26.4.

Please describe what you see

Figure 26.3 shows a hypermetabolic tumour spanning around 12.6cm in length at the oesophagus, corresponding to the endoscopic findings presented earlier. Figure 26.4 shows a hypermetabolic lymph node with calcification at the right hilar region up to 12.7cm in size, which is suggestive of nodal metastasis. (Other cuts also show likely nodal metastases to the right paratracheal and subcarinal regions.)

How would you manage this patient?

A multidisciplinary meeting with surgeons and oncologists should be held. In view of the metastatic disease, surgical treatment would unlikely benefit the patient. Also, the length of involvement is considered too extensive to consider radical radiotherapy. The overall plan is to consider palliative chemotherapy, and radiotherapy for symptomatic control. A self-expandable metallic stent is deployed to alleviate the symptoms of dysphagia (Figure 26.5).

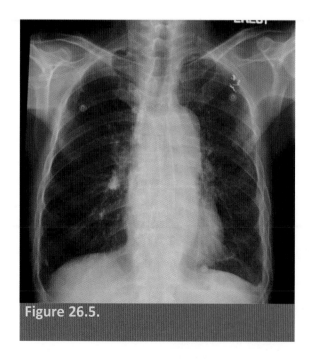

Figure 26.5.

Clinical pearls

- There are mainly two histological types of oesophageal carcinoma, namely squamous cell carcinoma (SCC) and adenocarcinoma. Worldwide, SCC is the most prevalent type, whereas in developed countries adenocarcinoma is more common.
- Risk factors for the development of SCC are:
  - alcohol [1];
  - smoking;
  - intake of preservatives containing nitrosamine;
  - Plummer-Vinson syndrome;
  - tylosis.
- Risk factors for the development of adenocarcinoma are:
  - gastrointestinal reflux disease;
  - Barrett's oesophagus [2];
  - obesity.

Impress your attending

What is the prognosis of oesophageal carcinoma?

As oesophageal carcinoma usually presents at an advanced stage, the overall prognosis is poor. Around 20-30% of patients at initial diagnosis will have distant metastasis [3]. Stage I disease has a 5-year survival of around 65%, compared with <5% with Stage IV disease.

What is trimodality therapy?

The use of neoadjuvant chemoradiation prior to surgery has been shown to improve survival [4, 5] (usually cisplatin and fluorouracil or carboplatin and paclitaxel [6]).

Are there any promising therapies on the horizon that you know of?

Immune checkpoint inhibition is a promising new therapeutic target for a multitude of advanced malignancies. In a recent phase 1b trial, the anti-programmed death-1 antibody, pembrolizumab, demonstrated manageable toxicity and durable anti-tumour activity in patients with heavily pretreated PD-L1-positive advanced oesophageal carcinoma [7].

References

1. Brown LM, Hoover RN, Greenberg RS, *et al.* Are racial differences in squamous cell esophageal cancer explained by alcohol and tobacco use? *J Natl Cancer Inst* 1994; 86: 1340-5.
2. Spechler SJ. Barrett esophagus and risk of esophageal cancer: a clinical review. *JAMA* 2013; 310: 627-36.
3. Quint LE, Hepburn LM, Francis IR, *et al.* Incidence and distribution of distant metastases from newly diagnosed esophageal carcinoma. *Cancer* 1995; 76: 1120-5.
4. Tepper J, Krasna MJ, Niedzwiecki D, *et al.* Phase III trial of trimodality therapy with cisplatin, fluorouracil, radiotherapy, and surgery compared with surgery alone for esophageal cancer: CALGB 9781. *J Clin Oncol* 2008; 26(7): 1086-92.
5. van Hagen P, Hulshof MC, van Lanschot JJ, *et al.* Preoperative chemoradiotherapy for esophageal or junctional cancer. *N Engl J Med* 2012; 366(22): 2074-84.
6. NCCN Clinical Practice Guidelines in Oncology, 2015. Esophageal and Esophagogastric Junction Cancers.
7. Doi T, Piha-Paul SA, Jalal SI, *et al.* Safety and antitumor activity of the anti-programmed death-1 antibody pembrolizumab in patients with advanced esophageal carcinoma. *J Clin Oncol* 2018; 36(1): 61-7.

Case 27

History

A 60-year-old lady presents with a longstanding history of dysphagia to both solids and liquids for several years. There is no odynophagia or weight loss. She did not seek any prior medical attention. Recently, she presents to the general medical ward with an episode of a severe chest infection.

Physical examination

- Temperature 38.5°C, pulse 120 bpm, BP 120/80mmHg, SaO$_2$ 98-100% on RA.
- Hydration is satisfactory.
- Examination of the hands reveals no clubbing and normal-appearing palmar creases.
- Head and neck examination is unremarkable.
- Cardiovascular: HS dual, no murmur.
- Auscultation of the chest reveals right lower zone crepitation.
- Abdominal examination reveals a soft, non-tender abdomen.
- No signs of oedema.

Investigations

- CBC — which reveals leukocytosis.
- Liver function tests are normal.
- Renal function tests are normal.
- Blood for culture to rule out septicaemia.

What is your differential diagnosis for her dysphagia?

- Achalasia.
- Chagas disease.
- Pseudoachalasia.

What other tests will you order?

- Sputum for culture and sensitivity.
- Chest X-ray for consolidative changes (Figure 27.1).

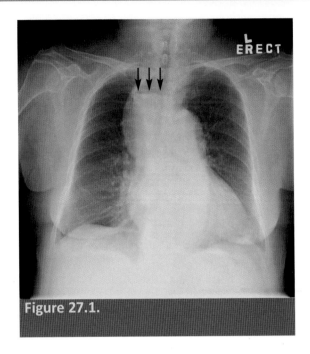

Figure 27.1.

Please describe what you see

A dilated tubular structure with an air-fluid level (arrows) is present in the mediastinum, which is suggestive of food residue in a dilated oesophagus.

How would you manage the acute medical condition?

- Keep the patient nil by mouth to prevent further aspiration.
- Start antibiotics with good anaerobic coverage.

After stabilisation, what would be the next investigation for her dysphagia?

Oesophagogastroduodenoscopy (OGD).

The OGD reveals a dilated oesophagus. No structural or mucosal abnormalities are identified.

What further investigation should be performed?

- Barium swallow. A barium swallow shows a 'bird's beak' appearance of the lower oesophageal sphincter (LOS) with incomplete opening.
- Oesophageal manometry (Figure 27.2).

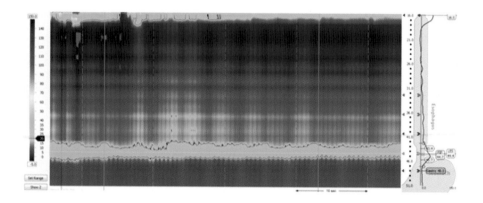

Figure 27.2.

Please describe what you see

High-resolution manometry (HRM) shows aperistalsis and the lower oesophageal sphincter failing to relax during swallowing.

What are the treatment options for achalasia?

The treatment of achalasia depends on the surgical risk [1]:

- Low surgical risk:
  - Heller myotomy or pneumatic dilatation (PD) [1];
  - peroral endoscopic myotomy (POEM) [2].
- High surgical risk:
  - medical therapy (e.g. nitrates or calcium channel blockers) [1];
  - pneumatic dilatation [1];
  - botulinum toxin injection [1].

Figure 27.3 is adapted from the American College of Gastroenterology (ACG) 2013 guideline — "Diagnosis and Management of Achalasia") [1].

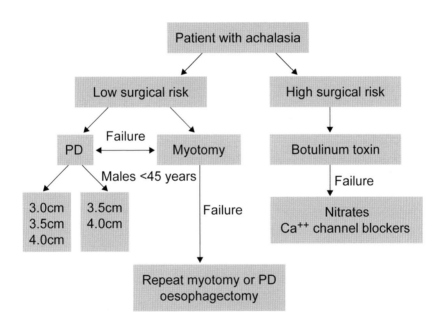

PD: pneumatic dilatation.

Figure 27.3. An algorithm for managing achalasia.

Clinical pearls

- Achalasia may present with dysphagia to both solids and liquids.
- Complications of achalasia include:
  - squamous cell carcinoma of the oesophagus (~1 cancer per 300 patient years) [3];
  - reflux oesophagitis [4];
  - megaoesophagus [4];
  - aspiration pneumonia [5];
  - malnutrition.
- Treatment of achalasia depends on the surgical risk of the patient.

Impress your attending

What are the causes of pseudoachalasia?
Psuedoachalasia may mimic achalasia clinically and manometrically [1].

Causes of pseudoachalasia include [1]:

- Mechanical obstruction from tumours in the gastric cardia.
- Tumours infiltrating the myenteric plexus (adenocarcinoma of the gastro-oesophageal junction, and pancreatic, breast, lung or hepatocellular cancers).
- Secondary achalasia from extrinsic processes such as a prior tight fundoplication or laparoscopic adjustable gastric banding.

What is POEM [2]?
- POEM stands for peroral endoscopic myotomy.
- It is done under general anaesthesia.

After submucosal injection, a mucosal incision is made 15cm above the gastro-oesophageal junction (GOJ) followed by submucosal tunnelling. A long submucosal tunnel is created to extend below the GOJ. The endoscopic myotomy starts 10cm above and extends 2cm below the GOJ. The mucosal entrance is closed with endoclips [2].

What is the performance of POEM compared with that of a Heller myotomy [6]?

POEM is associated with a shorter hospitalisation than a Heller myotomy.

Patient symptoms and oesophageal physiology are improved equally with both procedures.

Postoperative oesophageal acid exposure is the same for both.

References

1. Vaezi M, Pandolfino J, Vela M. Diagnosis and management of achalasia. *Am J Gastroenterol* 2013; 108: 1238-49.
2. Chiu PWY, Wu JCY, Teoh AY, *et al.* Peroral endoscopic myotomy for treatment of achalasia: from bench to bedside (with video). *Gastrointest Endosc* 2013; 77(1): 29-38.
3. Leeuwenburgh I, Scholten P, Alderliesten J, *et al.* Long-term esophageal cancer risk in patients with primary achalasia: a prospective study. *Am J Gastroenterol* 2010; 105: 2144-9.
4. Eckardt VF, Hoischen T, Bernhard G. Life expectancy, complications, and causes of death in patients with achalasia: results of a 33-year follow-up investigation. *Eur J Gastroenterol Hepatol* 2008; 20: 956-60.
5. O'Neill OM, Johnston BT, Coleman HG. Achalasia: a review of clinical diagnosis, epidemiology, treatment and outcomes. *World J Gastroenterol* 2013; 19(35): 5806-12.
6. Bhayani NH, Kurian AA, Dunst CM, *et al.* A comparative study on comprehensive, objective outcomes of laparoscopic Heller myotomy with per-oral endoscopic myotomy (POEM) for achalasia. *Ann Surg* 2014; 259(6): 1098-103.

Case 28

A 65-year-old lady with good past health presents to the emergency department with a 2-day history of fever, jaundice and right upper quadrant pain. On further questioning, she has experienced pain on and off over the last few months.

Physical examination

- Temperature 39°C, pulse 115 bpm, BP 90/50mmHg, SaO$_2$ 98-100% on RA.
- Slightly dehydrated, jaundice.
- Examination of the hands reveals no clubbing, normal-appearing palmar creases and warm peripheries.
- Head and neck examination is unremarkable.
- Cardiovascular: HS dual, no murmur.
- Her chest is clear on auscultation.
- Abdominal examination reveals a soft abdomen, with right upper quadrant tenderness. Murphy's sign is negative.
- No signs of oedema.

Investigations

- CBC:
  - WBC 19 x 10^9/L;
  - haemoglobin 12g/dL;
  - platelets 296 x 10^9/L.
- Total bilirubin 100μmol/L.
- ALP 412 IU/L.
- ALT 102 IU/L.
- Albumin 32g/L.
- Amylase normal.
- Blood culture to rule out septicaemia.
- CXR.
- ECG.

CXR shows no consolidative changes and no free gas under the diaphragm. ECG shows a normal sinus rhythm with no evidence of cardiac ischaemia.

What is your differential diagnosis?

- Acute cholangitis (most likely).
- Acute cholecystitis.
- Acute pancreatitis.
- Basal pneumonia.

What would you do next?

The initial treatment of cholangitis should consist of:

- Aggressive fluid resuscitation [1].
- Prompt initiation of intravenous antibiotics [1].
- Correction of coagulopathy [1].

IV vitamin K1 is given. After fluid resuscitation with 1.5L colloid and initiation of IV cefotaxime, the patient remains tachycardic with a heart rate of 110 bpm. Blood pressure is 100/50mmHg after fluid resuscitation. Urgent ultrasound is not available.

How would you proceed?

In view of severe cholangitis with haemodynamic instability despite fluid resuscitation and intravenous antibiotics, an urgent endoscopic retrograde cholangiopancreatography (ERCP) should be considered.

An urgent ERCP is performed after initial stabilisation.

Fluoroscopy shows the following (Figure 28.1).

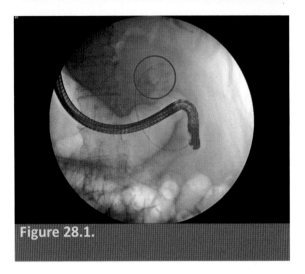

Figure 28.1.

Please describe what you see

This is a limited fluoroscopic image of an ERCP showing a dilated common bile duct and intrahepatic ducts with three stones of at least 2cm in size in the common bile duct.

How would you proceed endoscopically?

The primary focus of management at this juncture is immediate drainage rather than stone extraction [1, 2]:

- Injection of contrast medium under pressure should be avoided, as this may lead to cholangio-venous reflux and exacerbation of the septicaemia.
- Aspiration of infected bile before injecting contrast material may prevent the exacerbation of septicaemia.

Bile aspiration is done and sent for culture. A plastic stent is inserted with good bile drainage.

The patient becomes afebrile and liver function tests are normalised after ERCP. Bile and blood culture subsequently grow *Klebsiella pneumoniae.*

In view of septicaemia, the patient completes a 2-week course of antibiotics. A second ERCP is arranged for stone extraction.

Stone extraction is performed via a balloon extraction basket. A sphincterotomy is also performed. A final occlusion cholangiogram (OC) confirms the clearance of biliary ductal stones.

What would you do next?

An elective cholecystectomy should be arranged to prevent the recurrence of further complications of biliary stones [1, 3].

The timing of cholecystectomy is preferably done early (within 2 weeks) [1].

Studies have shown a higher morbidity and need for emergency surgery in patients receiving a delayed cholecystectomy as compared with the early group [4].

Clinical pearls

- Patients with cholangitis may not present with all three components of Charcot's triad (namely right upper quadrant pain, fever and jaundice). All three components are only seen in up to 70% of cases [5]. A high index of suspicion is required to avoid any delay in the diagnosis of acute cholangitis.
- The initial management of cholangitis includes aggressive fluid resuscitation, prompt initiation of antibiotics, correction of coagulopathy and early drainage of the biliary system.
- In patients with acute severe cholangitis, an initial ERCP aims at biliary decompression rather than stone removal.
- All patients with cholangitis due to stone disease should be referred for consideration of a cholecystectomy.

Impress your attending

What are the common organisms implicated in acute cholangitis [1]?
- *Pseudomonas aeruginosa.*
- *Enterobacter* species.
- *Bacteroides.*
- Fungal infections (e.g. *Candida*).

What are the treatment options for large biliary stones which fail conventional techniques?
- Lithotripsy involves procedures that fragment large stones, and they can be roughly classified into two groups: intracorporeal modalities and extracorporeal modalities [6].
- Intracorporeal modalities include:
  - mechanical lithotripsy (ML);
  - electrohydraulic lithotripsy;
  - laser lithotripsy.
- Extracorporeal modality:
  - extracorporeal shock-wave lithotripsy (ESWL).

How is mechanical lithotripsy performed?
- Large stones are captured in the lithotriptor basket [6].
- A metal sheath is advanced up to the level of the stone.
- Mechanical lithotripsy is performed by pulling the stone against the metal sleeve using a cranking device.
- Large stones are fragmented into multiple small pieces.
- An extraction basket can be used to remove these fragmented stones.

What is the limitation of mechanical lithotripsy?
Mechanical lithotripsy is less likely to be successful with larger and impacted stones [6].

How is electrohydraulic lithotripsy performed?
- An electrohydraulic shock-wave generator can fully pass through the working channel of the cholangioscope [6].

- A charge is transmitted across the electrodes at the tip of the probe and a spark is created.
- This induces expansion of the surrounding fluid and an oscillating spherical shock wave of a pressure sufficient to fragment the stone.
- Continuous saline irrigation is required to provide a media for shock-wave energy transmission, to ensure visualisation and to flush away debris.

How is cholangioscopic-guided laser lithotripsy performed?
- A sphincterotomy is performed to allow for the passage of the cholangioscope into the biliary tree [7].
- A fibreoptic probe and catheter system facilitates transpapillary access for the holmium laser.
- An aiming beam to target the stone and direct apposition can be confirmed via a cholangioscopic/pancreatoscopic view.
- Laser bursts of less than 5 seconds are delivered under continuous saline solution irrigation via the cholangioscopic irrigation channel.
- Stone fragmentation is deemed complete when fragments are no longer filling the lumen and are dispersed easily with fluid irrigation.

References

1. Bornman PC, van Beljon JI, Krige JEJ. Management of cholangitis. *J Hepatobiliary Pancreat Surg* 2003; 10: 406-14.
2. Lee DWH, Chung SCS. Biliary infection. *Baillière's Clin Gastroenterol* 1997; 11: 707-24.
3. McAlister VC, Davenport E, Renouf E. Cholecystectomy deferral in patients with endoscopic sphincterotomy. *Cochrane Database Syst Rev* 2007; 4: CD006233.
4. Reinders JS, Goud A, Timmer R, *et al.* Early laparoscopic cholecystectomy improves outcomes after endoscopic sphincterotomy for choledochocystolithiasis. *Gastroenterology* 2010; 138: 2315-20.

5. Stefanidis G, Christodoulou C, Manolakopoulos S, Chuttani R. Endoscopic extraction of large common bile duct stones: a review article. *World J Gastrointest Endosc* 2012; 4(5): 167.

6. Chan SS. How should biliary stones be managed? *Gut Liver* 2010; 4(2): 161-72.

7. Maydeo A, Kwek BEA, Bhandari S, *et al.* Single-operator cholangioscopy-guided laser lithotripsy in patients with difficult biliary and pancreatic ductal stones (with videos). *Gastrointest Endosc* 2011; 74(6): 1308-14.

Case 29

History

A 45-year-old lady with a history of bipolar affective disorder on long-term valproate presents to the emergency department with a 1-day history of severe epigastric pain radiating to the back. She describes the pain as sharp in nature with a pain score of 8 out of 10. She is a non-drinker.

Physical examination

- Temperature 37.5°C, pulse 115 bpm, BP 120/70mmHg, SaO$_2$ 98-100% on RA.
- Moderate dehydration.
- Examination of the hands reveals no clubbing, normal-appearing palmar creases and warm peripheries.
- Head and neck examination is unremarkable.
- Cardiovascular: HS dual, no murmur.
- Her chest is clear on auscultation.
- Abdominal examination reveals a soft abdomen, with moderate epigastric tenderness and no pulsatile mass. Murphy's sign is negative.
- No signs of oedema.

Investigations

- CBC:
    - WBC 17 x 10^9/L;
    - haemoglobin 12g/dL;
    - platelets 286 x 10^9/L.
- Total bilirubin 20µmol/L.
- ALP 47 IU/L.
- ALT 22 IU/L.
- Albumin 36g/L.
- Amylase 2130 IU/L.
- Creatinine 230µmol/L.
- Urea 15mmol/L.

What is your differential diagnosis?

- Acute pancreatitis (most likely).
- Ruptured/dissecting abdominal aortic aneurysm (AAA).
- Mesenteric ischaemia or infarction.
- Perforated gastric or duodenal ulcer.
- Biliary colic/cholecystitis.

What are the causes of elevated serum amylase [1]?

- Acute pancreatitis.
- Other pancreatic disease:
  - pancreatic pseudocyst;
  - pancreatic carcinoma.
- Biliary tract disease:
  - cholecystitis;
  - cholangitis.
- Intestinal obstruction, ischaemia or perforation.
- Acute appendicitis.
- Renal failure.
- Macroamylasaemia.
- Gynaecological disease: ovarian tumour, ectopic pregnancy.
- Diabetic ketoacidosis.

How would you make a diagnosis of acute pancreatitis?

The diagnosis of acute pancreatitis is made with any two out of the three following criteria [2]:

- Abdominal pain consistent with the disease.
- Serum amylase or lipase >3x upper limit.
- Characteristic findings from abdominal imaging.

What are the causes of acute pancreatitis [1]?

- Biliary:
  - gallstones;
  - microlithiasis.
- Alcohol.
- Anatomic variants:
  - pancreas divisum;
  - choledochal cyst;
  - duodenal duplication;

- santorinicoele;
- duodenal diverticula.
- Mechanical obstructions to the flow of pancreatic juice:
  - ampullary: benign and malignant tumours, stricture or dysfunction of the sphincter of Oddi;
  - ductal: stones, strictures, masses (including tumours), mucus (e.g. in intraductal papillary mucinous neoplasms), parasites (*Ascaris*).
- Metabolic:
  - hypercalcaemia;
  - hypertriglyceridaemia.
- Drugs (including valproate [3]).
- Toxins.
- Trauma:
  - blunt and penetrating;
  - instrumentation (ERCP, pancreatic biopsy).
- Ischaemia:
  - hypotension;
  - arteritis;
  - embolic.
- Hypothermia.
- Infections:
  - viral (mumps, Coxsackie A, human immunodeficiency virus);
  - bacterial/other (*M. tuberculosis*, *Mycoplasma*);
  - parasites (*Ascaris*);
  - venoms (spider, Gila monster).
- Autoimmune.
- Genetic (familial, sporadic).
- Idiopathic.

How would you further investigate the patient to elucidate the aetiology?

- Fasting lipid profile (for hypertriglyceridaemia) [2].
- Ultrasound (USG) abdomen (for gallstone disease) [2].

A USG of the abdomen does not reveal any gallstones. The fasting lipid profile is normal. The likely aetiology of pancreatitis is valproate and it is stopped.

Further testing shows the following:

- Random glucose on admission was 12mmol/L.
- Serum aspartate aminotransferase level (AST) 170 IU/L.
- Serum lactate dehydrogenase level (LDH) 400 IU/L.
- Haematocrit 0.383.

Blood tests 48 hours after admission show the following:

- Serum calcium 2.1mmol/L.
- Haematocrit 0.351.
- Arterial pO_2 80mmHg.
- Urea 15mmol/L.
- Base deficit -6.

Clinically, the patient is dehydrated and estimated sequestration of fluid is 8L.

Calculate the Ranson score of this patient

The Ranson score is measured in two stages: 5 initial data points on admission and a further 6 data points within the subsequent 48 hours [4]. (The patient's scores are shown in brackets below.)

On admission:

- Age >55 (0).
- White cell count >16 cells/mm^3 (1).
- Serum glucose >10mmol/L (1).
- Serum lactate dehydrogenase (LDH) level >350 IU/L (1).
- Serum aspartate aminotransferase (AST) level >250 IU/L (0).

48 hours after admission:

- Calcium <2.0mmol/L (0).

- Decrease in haematocrit by >10% (1).
- Hypoxaemia pO_2 <60mmHg (0).
- Blood urea nitrogen level increase by 1.8 or more mmol/L after IV fluid (0).
- Base deficit >4mEq/L (1).
- Sequestration of fluid >6L (1).

The total score for this patient is 6 (a score of 3 is predictive of severe acute pancreatitis).

The patient is managed in the intensive care unit (ICU). Aggressive fluid resuscitation and oxygen therapy are given. Enteral feeding is continued. Her renal function continues to deteriorate and continuous veno-venous haemofiltration (CVVH) is started for renal support. Five days after admission, she develops a spike of fever.

A contrast CT abdomen is performed (Figure 29.1).

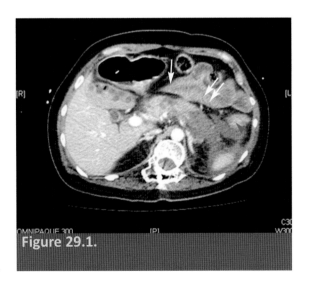

Figure 29.1.

Please describe what you see

The pancreas is diffusely enlarged with patchy non-enhancing areas (white arrows) suggestive of necrosis in the neck, body and tail.

Moderate peripancreatic stranding and fluid (arrowhead) are noted.

No pancreatic ductal dilatation or abnormal calcification is seen.

How would you manage this patient?

This patient is suffering from infected pancreatic necrosis. Empirical antibiotics with good pancreatic penetration (e.g. carbapenem) should be started [2].

Prompt surgical treatment should be offered if the patient becomes unstable [2].

The patient is treated with meropenem. However, she continues to deteriorate and a surgical necrosectomy is performed. She remains stable after a necrosectomy. Valproate is stopped. She remains well and there is no recurrence of pancreatitis.

Clinical pearls

- The diagnosis of acute pancreatitis is made with any two out of the three following criteria:
  - abdominal pain consistent with the disease;
  - serum amylase or lipase >3x the upper limit;
  - characteristic findings from abdominal imaging.
- Pancreatic necrosis is one possible complication of acute pancreatitis.
- Infected pancreatic necrosis should be treated by antibiotics with good pancreatic penetration (e.g. carbapenem) and prompt surgical treatment should be offered if the patient becomes unstable.

Impress your attending

What is the predictive value of the Ranson score?

A Ranson score of >3 predicts severe acute pancreatitis as follows [5]:

- Sensitivity 75%.
- Specificity of 77%.
- Positive predictive value 49%.
- Negative predictive value 91%.

How would you classify acute pancreatitis?

The revised Atlanta Classification updated in 2012 [6] defines various morphological features of acute pancreatitis:

- According to contrast-enhancing CT criteria, acute pancreatitis can be divided into:
  - interstitial oedematous pancreatitis;
  - necrotising pancreatitis (5-10% of patients).
- The nomenclature for local complications has also been revised — see Table 29.1.

Table 29.1. Revised nomenclature for local complications of pancreatitis.	
<4 weeks	**>4 weeks**
Acute peripancreatic fluid collection (APFC)	**Pancreatic pseudocyst**
• Sterile	• Sterile
• Infected	• Infected
Acute necrotic collection (ANC)	**Pancreatic walled-off necrosis (PWON)**
• Sterile	• Sterile
• Infected	• Infected

References

1. Forsmark CE, Baillie J. AGA Institute technical review on acute pancreatitis. *Gastroenterology* 2007; 132(5): 2022-44.
2. Tenner S, Baillie J, DeWitt J, *et al.* American College of Gastroenterology guideline: management of acute pancreatitis. *Am J Gastroenterol* 2013; 108(9): 1400-15.
3. Gerstner T, Büsing D, Bell N, *et al.* Valproic acid-induced pancreatitis: 16 new cases and a review of the literature. *J Gastroenterol* 2007; 42(1): 39-48.
4. Ranson JH, Rifkind KM, Roses DF, *et al.* Prognostic signs and the role of operative management in acute pancreatitis. *Surgery, Gynecology & Obstetrics* 1974; 139(1): 69-81.
5. Larvin M. Assessment of clinical severity and prognosis. In: Beger HG, Warshaw AL, Buchler MW, *et al*, Eds. *The Pancreas*. Oxford, UK: Blackwell Science, 1998: 489-502.
6. Banks PA, Bollen TL, Dervenis C, *et al*; Acute Pancreatitis Classification Working Group. Classification of acute pancreatitis - 2012: revision of the Atlanta classification and definitions by international consensus. *Gut* 2013; 62(1): 102-11.

Case 30

A 76-year-old gentleman presents to the outpatient clinic with a 2-month history of jaundice associated with dark-coloured urine. He has no fever, abdominal pain or weight loss. He has a history of hypertension, hyperlipidaemia and chronic obstructive airway disease. He is taking nifedipine and simvastatin but there has been no recent change in dosage. He is a non-drinker and denies use of over-the-counter medications or herbs.

Physical examination

- Temperature 36.7°C, pulse 75 bpm, BP 135/80mmHg, SaO_2 98-100% on RA.
- Hydration good, with jaundice.
- Examination of the hands reveals no clubbing and normal-appearing palmar creases.
- Head and neck examination is unremarkable.
- Cardiovascular: HS dual. No murmur.
- His chest is clear on auscultation.
- Abdominal examination reveals a soft, non-tender abdomen, with a vague palpable mass at the right upper quadrant.
- No signs of oedema.

Investigations

- CBC:
  - WBC 8 x 10^9/L;
  - haemoglobin 13.5g/dL;
  - platelets 298 x 10^9/L.
- Total bilirubin 65μmol/L.
- ALP 412 IU/L.
- ALT 78 IU/L.
- Albumin 38g/L.

What is the differential diagnosis of jaundice?

Increased unconjugated bilirubin:

- Increased bilirubin production.
- Haemolytic anaemia.
- Ineffective haemopoiesis.
- Gilbert's syndrome (less likely given the extent of hyperbilirubinaemia).

Increased conjugated bilirubin:

- Hepatocellular disease.
- Intrahepatic and extrahepatic biliary obstruction.
- Total parenteral nutrition.

What is the pattern of liver function abnormality?

An obstructive pattern (predominant increase in ALP).

Does this narrow down your differential diagnosis?

Biliary obstruction is more likely.

The causes of biliary obstruction include:

- Intraductal:
  - biliary stones;
  - biliary flukes;
  - haemobilia.
- Ductal:
  - cholangiocarcinoma;
  - cholangiopathy (including primary sclerosing cholangitis);
  - primary biliary cirrhosis;
  - choledochal cyst.
- Extraductal:
  - pancreatic head mass;
  - ampullary lesion;
  - enlarged lymph nodes in the porta hepatis.

What is Courvoisier's law?

Courvoisier's law states that in the presence of an enlarged gallbladder which is non-tender and accompanied with mild jaundice, the cause is unlikely to be gallstones [1].

What are the exceptions to Courvoisier's law?

The exceptions to the law are stones that dislodge and acutely jam the duct distally to the hepatic/cystic duct junction:

- Gallstone falling and blocking the Ampulla of Vater.
- Gallstone falling and blocking the cystic/hepatic duct junction.
- Double impaction by stones.

What further imaging would you order?

Ultrasound (USG) of the abdomen.

USG of the abdomen is performed showing a dilated common bile duct (CBD) sized at 1.2cm with bilateral dilated intrahepatic ducts (IHD). There are no gallstones or biliary stones. The visualised part of the pancreas appears unremarkable.

Endoscopic retrograde cholangiopancreatography (ERCP) is performed. An endoscopic view (Figure 30.1) and fluoroscopy (Figure 30.2) shows the following.

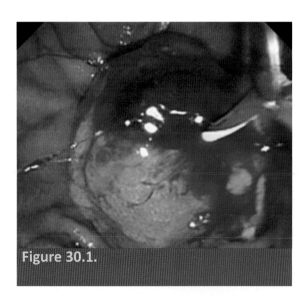

Figure 30.1.

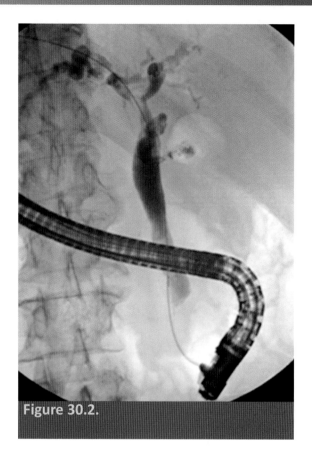

Figure 30.2.

Please describe what you see

The endoscopic view shows an ampullary mass. The fluoroscopic image shows a dilated CBD and IHD with no obvious filling defects.

Biopsy of the ampullary mass shows adenomatous proliferation with mild dysplasia.

What condition is associated with ampullary adenoma?

Familial adenomatous polyposis (FAP) is associated with ampullary adenoma [2, 3].

How would you proceed further regarding the management of the ampullary adenoma?

Endoscopic ultrasound (EUS) should be arranged.

EUS can provide information regarding the depth of the ampullary lesion as well as locoregional lymph node status [4].

Multiple studies have shown that EUS is superior to CT, MRI and transabdominal US in local peri-ampullary tumour staging [4].

EUS is arranged showing a 2cm hypoechoic ampullary adenoma and CBD dilation to 1.7cm. The pancreatic duct is not dilated. There is no locoregional lymph node enlargement.

Endoscopic resection of the adenoma is performed. One-year surveillance duodenoscopy shows no recurrence.

Clinical pearls

- Ampullary adenoma is a cause of biliary obstruction.
- Endoscopic resection is a possible treatment option for properly selected ampullary neoplasms.
- FAP is associated with ampullary adenoma.

Impress your attending

What is the success rate of endoscopic papillectomy for ampullary adenoma?
Success rates for endoscopic removal of ampullary adenomas range from 46% to 92%. Recurrence rates range from 0% to 33% [5].

What are the factors predicting the success of papillectomy?
Smaller lesion size and the absence of dilated ducts are factors favourable for success [6].

Jaundice at presentation, occult adenocarcinoma in the resected specimen, and intraductal involvement are associated with a lower rate of complete resection [7].

As recurrence has been observed up to 5 years after resection, long-term surveillance is warranted.

References

1. Parmar MS. Courvoisier's law. *CMAJ* 2003; 168(7): 876-7.
2. Heiskanen I, Kellokumpu I, Järvinen H. Management of duodenal adenomas in 98 patients with familial adenomatous polyposis. *Endoscopy* 1999; 31(6): 412.
3. Offerhaus GJ, Giardiello FM, Krush AJ, *et al.* The risk of upper gastrointestinal cancer in familial adenomatous polyposis. *Gastroenterology* 1992; 102(6): 1980.
4. Chini P, Draganov PV. Diagnosis and management of ampullary adenoma: the expanding role of endoscopy. *World J Gastrointest Endosc* 2011; 3(12): 241.
5. Han J, Kim MH. Endoscopic papillectomy for adenomas of the major duodenal papilla (with video). *Gastrointest Endosc* 2006; 63: 292-301.
6. Irani S, Arai A, Ayub K, *et al.* Papillectomy for ampullary neoplasm: results of a single referral center over a 10-year period. *Gastrointest Endosc* 2009; 70: 923-32.
7. Ridtitid W, Tan D, Schmidt SE, *et al.* Endoscopic papillectomy: risk factors for incomplete resection and recurrence during long-term follow-up. *Gastrointest Endosc* 2014; 79(2): 289-96.

Case 31

History

A 52-year-old lady with a longstanding history of gastro-oesophageal reflux disease (GORD) presents with a recent increase in epigastric discomfort and heartburn. She has no tarry stools, haematemesis, dysphagia or weight loss. She has a body mass index of 28kg/m².

Physical examination

- Temperature 36.5°C, fever, pulse 80 bpm, BP 120/80mmHg, SaO_2 98-100% on RA.
- Obese, hydration satisfactory.
- Examination of the hands reveals no clubbing and normal-appearing palmar creases.
- Head and neck examination is unremarkable.
- Cardiovascular: HS dual, no murmur.
- Her chest is clear on auscultation.
- Abdominal examination reveals a soft, non-tender abdomen.
- No signs of oedema.

Investigations

- CBC:
  - WBC 5 x 10^9/L;
  - haemoglobin 12.5g/dL;
  - platelets 278 x 10^9/L.

What is your differential diagnosis?

- GORD.
- Malignancy (e.g. liver, oesophageal, gastric).
- Drugs (all non-steroidal anti-inflammatory drugs [NSAIDs]).
- Pancreatic disease (chronic pancreatitis).
- Gastroparesis.
- Functional dyspepsia.

Would you arrange an oesophagogastroduodenoscopy (OGD) for this patient?

Yes. Patients with a new onset of dyspepsia after 45 to 55 years of age and those with alarming symptoms should undergo an initial endoscopy [1].

Alarming features include [1]:

- Family history of upper-GI malignancy.

- Unintended weight loss.
- GI bleeding or iron deficiency anaemia.
- Progressive dysphagia.
- Odynophagia.
- Persistent vomiting.
- Palpable mass or lymphadenopathy.
- Jaundice.

An OGD is performed showing the following (Figure 31.1).

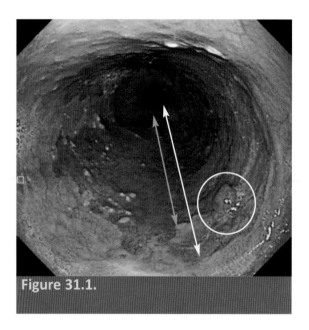

Figure 31.1.

Please describe what you see

White light endoscopy shows no oesophagitis. The salmon-coloured mucosa noted above the oesophagogastric junction (OGJ) is suggestive of Barrett's oesophagus. A 5mm nodule (circle) is noted in the area of Barrett's oesophagus.

Upon endoscopic measurement, the diaphragmatic level is at 36cm and the OGJ is at 34cm. The salmon-coloured mucosa is noted at 29cm (highest point — white arrow) and 30cm (circumferential — blue arrow) to 34cm.

How would you report the Prague classification in this case?

The Prague classification is the extent of circumferential columnar-appearing mucosa above the OGJ, reported as the C value (4cm in this case), while the maximum extent of any tongue-like areas of columnar-appearing mucosa above the OGJ is reported as the M value (5cm in this case) [2]. Therefore, the Prague classification in this case should be reported as C4M5.

How would you take biopsies?

Four-quadrant biopsy specimens should be taken every 2cm [3].

In addition, special attention and targeted biopsies should be focused on lesions such as nodules, ulcers, and other mucosal irregularities because these lesions are more likely to demonstrate dysplasia or cancer [3].

Biopsies reveal Barrett's oesophagus with high-grade dysplasia.

Endoscopic ultrasound (EUS) is arranged. There is submucosal invasion of the nodule but there are no obvious enlarged peri-oesophageal lymph nodes (LN), celiac LN, or mediastinal LN.

How would you further manage the patient?

Endoscopic mucosal resection (EMR) should be offered for the visible mucosal irregularity.

EMR is performed. Histology shows high-grade glandular dysplasia on a background of Barrett's oesophagus. There is no definite stromal invasion or lymphovascular permeation and the resection margin is clear.

Clinical pearls

- In patients presenting with dyspepsia, an endoscopic work-up should be offered if the patient has alarming features.
- Endoscopic findings of Barrett's oesophagus are reported by the Prague classification.
- Four-quadrant biopsy specimens should be taken every 2cm and additional targeted biopsies at suspicious areas should be performed in patients with Barrett's oesophagus.

Impress your attending

What is the definition of Barrett's oesophagus?

Barrett's oesophagus is a change in the distal oesophageal epithelium of any length that can be recognised as columnar-type mucosa at endoscopy and is confirmed to have intestinal metaplasia by biopsy of the tubular oesophagus [3].

Is universal screening for Barrett's oesophagus recommended? If not, who should be screened?

Universal screening of Barrett's oesophagus is not recommended in the general population with GORD [4].

Screening can be considered on an individual basis in those who have multiple risk factors [4, 5].

Risk factors for Barrett's oesophagus include: age older than 50 years, male sex, white race, chronic GORD, hiatal hernia, elevated body mass index, and intra-abdominal distribution of body fat [4].

Would the presence of oesophagitis affect your management in a patient with Barrett's oesophagus?

Ideally, erosive oesophagitis should be healed prior to biopsy to increase the yield; this is to avoid missing short segments of columnar lining (oesophagitis may mask Barrett's oesophagus); 12% may have Barrett's oesophagus after healing of oesophagitis.

On the other hand, inflammation may be mistaken as low-grade dysplasia. Therefore, it is best to perform OGD again when the oesophagitis is healed.

Is surveillance endoscopy recommended for patients with confirmed Barrett's oesophagus?

The recommended surveillance interval for patients with confirmed Barrett's oesophagus from the American College of Gastroenterology (ACG) and American Gastroenterological Association (AGA) are outlined in Table 31.1.

Table 31.1. The recommended surveillance interval for patients with confirmed Barrett's oesophagus from the American College of Gastroenterology (ACG) and American Gastroenterological Association (AGA).

	ACG [3]	AGA [4]
No dysplasia	3-year intervals	3-5-year intervals
Mild dysplasia	Every 6 months x 2; then every 12 months	6-12-month intervals
Severe dysplasia	3-month intervals if the patient does not receive endoscopic therapy	3-month intervals if the patient does not receive endoscopic therapy

What is the risk for cancer in patients with high-grade dysplasia in Barrett's oesophagus?

High-grade dysplasia is associated with a 30% risk of cancer development [3].

How would you manage patients who have biopsy-confirmed Barrett's oesophagus with high-grade dysplasia?

- High-grade dysplasia, after confirmation from two pathologists, represents the threshold for treatment [3].

- Treatment options include: endoscopic mucosal resection (EMR), photodynamic therapy, radio-frequency ablation (RFA) [3].

What is the role of EMR in the treatment of high-grade dysplasia in Barrett's oesophagus after EUS assessment?

Standard EUS accurately predicts the depth of invasion for early oesophageal cancers in only 50% to 60% of cases [6].

EMR is a minimally invasive treatment for high-grade dysplasia and early oesophageal adenocarcinoma in Barrett's oesophagus and can provide additional useful information for staging of focal nodules [7].

References

1. Ikenberry SO, Harrison ME, Lichtenstein D, *et al*. The role of endoscopy in dyspepsia. *Gastrointest Endosc* 2007; 66: 1071-5.
2. Sharma P, Dent J, Armstrong D, *et al*. The development and validation of an endoscopic grading system for Barrett's esophagus: the Prague C & M criteria. *Gastroenterology* 2006; 131: 1392-9.
3. Wang KK, Sampliner RE; Practice Parameters Committee of the American College of Gastroenterology. Updated guidelines 2008 for the diagnosis, surveillance and therapy of Barrett's esophagus. *Am J Gastroenterol* 2008; 103: 788-97.
4. American Gastroenterological Association Guideline on Barrett's Esophagus. Published online March 5, 2014.
5. ASGE Standards of Practice Committee; Evans JA, Early DS, Fukami N, *et al*. The role of endoscopy in Barrett's esophagus and other premalignant conditions of the esophagus. *Gastrointest Endosc* 2012; 76: 1087-94.
6. Falk GW, Catalano MF, Sivak MV Jr, *et al*. Endosonography in the evaluation of patients with Barrett's esophagus and high-grade dysplasia. *Gastrointest Endosc* 1994; 40: 207-12.
7. Larghi A, Lightdale CJ, Memeo L, *et al*. EUS followed by EMR for staging of high-grade dysplasia and early cancer in Barrett's esophagus. *Gastrointest Endosc* 2005; 62(1): 16-23.

Case 32

A 47-year-old gentleman with a history of asthma on inhaled glucocorticoids presents with odynophagia of 2-month onset. He has no definite dysphagia and can tolerate an oral diet. He has no weight loss or other constitutional symptoms.

Physical examination

- Temperature 37.1°C, pulse 66 bpm, BP 108/68mmHg, SaO_2 98-100% on RA.
- Alert, no jaundice.
- Examination of the hands reveals no clubbing and normal-appearing palmar creases.
- Head and neck examination is unremarkable.
- Cardiovascular: HS dual, no murmur.
- His chest is clear on auscultation.
- Abdominal examination is normal.
- Oral exam: oral thrush present.
- No signs of oedema.

Investigations

- CBC:
    - WBC 7.4 x 10^9/L;
    - haemoglobin 12g/dL;
    - platelets 276 x 10^9/L.

What is the differential diagnosis?

Infective causes:

- *Cytomegalovirus.*
- Gingivitis.
- *Herpes simplex* virus.
- Pharyngitis (sore throat).
- Candidiasis.

Motility causes:

- Achalasia.
- Oesophageal spasms.
- Nutcracker oesophagus.

Others:

- Drug-induced oesophageal ulcers.
- Inflammatory conditions (e.g. Crohn's disease, Behçet's disease).
- Foreign body ingestion.

How would you investigate the patient further?

Oesophagogastroduodenoscopy (OGD).

An OGD is performed (Figure 32.1).

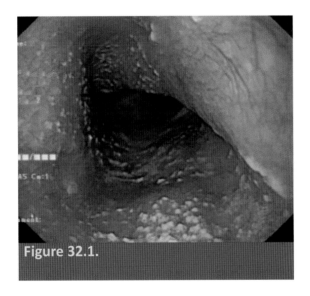

Figure 32.1.

Please describe what you see
There are multiple whitish plaque-like lesions noted on the oesophageal mucosa.

What is the most likely diagnosis?

Oesophageal candidiasis.

How would you manage this patient?

Systemic antifungal therapy.

Oral fluconazole is given for 2 weeks. Repeated endoscopy in 2 months reveals no more candidiasis.

How would you advise your patient to reduce the risk of recurrence of oesophageal candidiasis?

If possible, to reduce the daily dose of inhaled steroid [1]. The patient should be advised to rinse his mouth after steroid puffs.

Clinical pearls

- The use of inhaled steroids is associated with oesophageal candidiasis.
- Oral thrush has a good positive predictive value of oesophageal candidiasis in immunosuppressed patients [2].
- White or yellowish mucosal plaque-like lesions are the typical appearance of oesophageal candidiasis on OGD [3].
- Oesophageal candidiasis should be treated with systemic fluconazole [4].

Impress your attending

What is the predictive value of oral candidiasis for oesophageal candidiasis in immunocompromised patients?

The positive and negative predictive values of oropharyngeal candidiasis for oesophageal candidiasis are 90% and 82%, respectively [2].

What is the prevalence of oesophageal candidiasis among patients treated with inhaled corticosteroids?

The prevalence of oesophageal candidiasis was 37% among patients treated with inhaled fluticasone propionate [1].

The prevalence was especially high among patients with diabetes mellitus or those who were treated with a high dose of inhaled fluticasone propionate [1].

References

1. Kanda N, Yasuba H, Takahashi T, *et al.* Prevalence of esophageal candidiasis among patients treated with inhaled fluticasone propionate. *Am J Gastroenterol* 2003; 98: 2146-9.
2. Darouiche RO. Oropharyngeal and esophageal candidiasis in immunocompromised patients: treatment issues. *Clin Infect Dis* 1998; 26(2): 259-72.
3. Pech O. Esophageal candidiasis. *Video Journal and Encyclopedia of Gastrointest Endosc* 2013; 1(1): 64-5.
4. Pappas PG, Kauffman CA, Andes D, *et al.* Clinical practice guidelines for the management of candidiasis: 2009 update by the Infectious Diseases Society of America. *Clin Infect Dis* 2009; 48(5): 503-35.

Case 33

History

A 66-year-old gentleman with good past health presents with a 2-year history of steatorrhoea. He describes loose and foul-smelling stools that are difficult to flush. He also complains of epigastric pain. There is no weight loss. He is a chronic smoker and has drunk up to 5 cans of beer each day for the past 40 years. He is not on any medications. He also denies using over-the-counter drugs.

Physical examination

- Temperature 36.8°C, pulse 72 bpm, BP 133/78mmHg, SaO_2 98-100% on RA.
- Hydration satisfactory, alcoholic smell.
- Examination of the hands reveals no clubbing, normal-appearing palmar creases and warm peripheries.
- Head and neck examination is unremarkable.
- Cardiovascular: HS dual, no murmur.
- His chest is clear on auscultation.
- Abdominal examination reveals a soft abdomen, with mild epigastric tenderness. Murphy's sign is negative.
- No signs of oedema.

Investigations

- CBC:
  - WBC 9 x 10^9/L;
  - haemoglobin 13g/dL;
  - platelets 304 x 10^9/L.
- Total bilirubin 12µmol/L.
- ALP 35 IU/L.
- ALT 102 IU/L.
- Albumin 30g/L.
- Amylase normal.

What is your differential diagnosis?

- Chronic pancreatitis.
- Biliary obstruction.
- Peptic ulcer disease.
- Irritable bowel syndrome.
- Small bowel bacterial overgrowth.
- Celiac disease.

What further investigations would you perform?

- Abdominal X-ray.
- CT abdomen with contrast.
- Fasting glucose and HbA1C.

His fasting glucose is 13. A CT of the abdomen with contrast is performed (Figure 33.1).

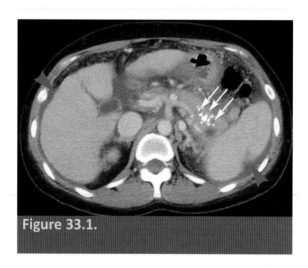

Figure 33.1.

Please describe what you see
The pancreas is slightly small in size.

Multiple calcific foci are present in the body and tail of the pancreas (arrows).

No focal pancreatic mass or pancreatic ductal dilatation is present.

There is a small amount of ascites present (arrowheads).

What is the most likely diagnosis?

Chronic pancreatitis.

What are the causes of chronic pancreatitis [1]?

- Ductal obstruction:
  - biliary stone;
  - tumour;
  - trauma;
  - pancreatic divisum.
- Toxin/metabolic:
  - alcohol;
  - hypercalcaemia;
  - hypertriglyceridaemia;
  - chronic renal failure;
  - drugs: valproate, phenacetin, thiazide, oestrogen and azathioprine;
  - infection: HIV, mumps virus, Coxsackie virus, *Echinococcus*, *Cryptosporidium*.
- Systemic disease:
  - vascular disease;
  - cystic fibrosis.
- Autoimmune.
- Genetic cause.
- Idiopathic.

What further testing would you perform to find out the aetiology?

- Serum calcium level.
- Fasting lipid profile.
- Renal function test (RFT).
- Ultrasound (USG) of the abdomen.

The RFT, serum calcium and fasting triglyceride are normal. The USG of the abdomen is unremarkable with no biliary gallstones seen. Given the history of the patient, the most likely aetiology of chronic pancreatitis in this patient is alcohol.

How would you manage the patient?

- General:
  - alcohol cessation [1];
  - stop smoking [1];
  - frequent small meals to limit pancreatic enzyme secretion and to reduce symptoms of maldigestion.
- Pain control [1, 2]:
  - NSAID;
  - adjunct therapy, e.g. pregabalin, tricyclic antidepressant;
  - endoscopic dilatation or stenting of the pancreatic duct;
  - surgery.
- Treatment of steatorrhoea [1]:
  - 30,000 IU of lipase per meal in an acid-resistant enzyme preparation.
- Treatment of diabetes mellitus [1]:
  - insulin therapy is required.
- Treatment of complications, if present [1]:
  - e.g. drainage of pseudocyst.

Clinical pearls

- Recurrent abdominal pain and steatorrhoea are two common presenting symptoms of chronic pancreatitis.
- Treatment of chronic pancreatitis should include alcohol and smoking cessation, treatment of pain and steatorrhoea, and treatment of complications.
- Hypoglycaemia is common in patients with chronic pancreatitis complicated with diabetes.

Impress your attending

Which of the causes of chronic pancreatitis are associated with pancreatic calcifications?
- Alcoholic pancreatitis.
- Tropical chronic pancreatitis [3].

Why is hypoglycaemia common in patients with chronic pancreatitis?
Both glucagon and insulin production is impaired in chronic pancreatitis.

How should chronic pancreatitis associated with a dominant stricture of the main pancreatic duct be managed?
The stricture should be managed with a single 10-Fr plastic stent, with stent exchange planned within 1 year [4].

In patients with ductal strictures persisting after 12 months of single plastic stenting, endoscopic placement of multiple pancreatic stents or surgery may be considered.

How should pancreatic stones associated with chronic pancreatitis be managed?
Extracorporeal shock wave lithotripsy (ESWL) or endoscopic retrograde cholangiopancreatography (ERCP) are the first-line interventional options.

If the clinical response at 6-8 weeks is unsatisfactory, a surgical option may be considered.

References

1. Braganza JM, Lee SH, McCloy RF, McMahon MJ. Chronic pancreatitis. *Lancet* 2011; 377(9772): 1184-97.
2. Forsmark CE. Management of chronic pancreatitis. *Gastroenterology* 2013; 144(6): 1282-91.

3. Barman KK, Premalatha G, Mohan V. Tropical chronic pancreatitis. *Postgrad Med J* 2003; 79: 606-15.

4. Dumonceau J-M, Delhaye M, Tringali A, *et al.* Endoscopic treatment of chronic pancreatitis: European Society of Gastrointestinal Endoscopy (ESGE) clinical guideline. *Endoscopy* 2012; 44(8): 784.

Case 34

A 45-year-old gentleman read about colorectal cancer screening in a local newspaper. He is asymptomatic and has no history of per rectal bleeding, change of bowel habits or constitutional symptoms. He is a smoker and is obese with a body mass index (BMI) of 28kg/m^2. He has a past history of non-alcoholic fatty liver disease. His brother died of colorectal cancer at the age of 54. He attends your clinic for advice on colorectal cancer screening. Physical examination is unremarkable.

Physical examination

- Afebrile, pulse 80 bpm, BP 120/80mmHg, SaO_2 98-100% on RA.
- Hydration is satisfactory.
- Examination of the hands reveals no clubbing and normal-appearing palmar creases.
- Head and neck examination is unremarkable.
- Cardiovascular: HS dual, no murmur.
- His chest is clear on auscultation.
- Abdominal examination reveals a soft, non-tender abdomen, with no peritoneal signs.
- No signs of oedema.

Investigations

- CBC:
  - WBC 9 x 10^9/L;
  - haemoglobin 13.5g/dL;
  - platelets 304 x 10^9/L.
- Liver and renal function tests are normal.

What are the risk factors for colorectal neoplasm in this patient?

- Male gender [1].
- Positive family history [1].
- Cigarette smoking [1].
- Obesity [1].
- Fatty liver disease [2].

In general, when should colorectal cancer screening commence?

- A diagnostic work-up should be commenced immediately in symptomatic patients [1].
- In asymptomatic patients, the timing for starting screening depends on the risk.

- Average-risk group:
  - screening begins at age 50 years [1];
  - screening begins at age 45 years in African Americans [1].
- Positive family history:
  - one first-degree relative affected at age ≥60 [3]:
    - average-risk screening but beginning at age 40 [1];
  - two or more first-degree relatives affected or one first-degree relative affected at age <60:
    - colonoscopy beginning age 40 or 10 years earlier than the youngest diagnosis in the family, whichever is earlier [1];
  - hereditary non-polyposis colorectal cancer (HNPCC): age 20 to 25 or 10 years before the youngest case in the immediate family [4];
  - familial adenomatous polyposis (FAP): age 10 to 12 [4].

An algorithm for colorectal cancer screening is outlined in Figure 34.1.

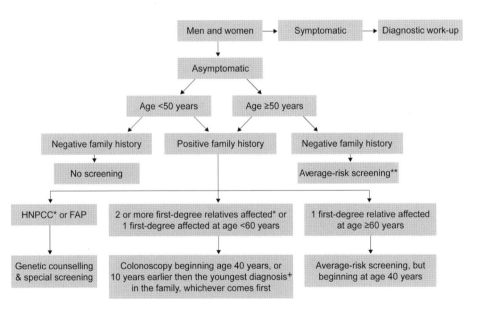

+ Either colorectal cancer or adenomatous polyp.
* HNPCC: hereditary non-polyposis colorectal cancer.
** See text.
FAP: familial adenomatous polyposis.

Figure 34.1. An algorithm for colorectal cancer screening.

What are the sensitivities of colorectal cancer screening tests?

The sensitivities of colorectal cancer screening tests are tabulated below (Table 34.1 [5-7]).

Table 34.1. Comparison of various colorectal cancer screening tests.

	Sensitivity %	
	Colorectal cancer	Advanced adenoma
Guaiac FOB	50-75	20-25
Immunochemical FOB	60-85	20-50
Barium enema	50	48
CT colonography	Uncertain ~>90	>90 (if >10mm)
Sigmoidoscopy	~70	70
Colonoscopy	>95	88-98

FOB: faecal occult blood.

In view of the positive family history with one first-degree relative affected at age <60, screening is offered. What screening test would you recommend for this patient?

Colonoscopy should be offered [1].

Colonoscopy is performed (Figure 34.2).

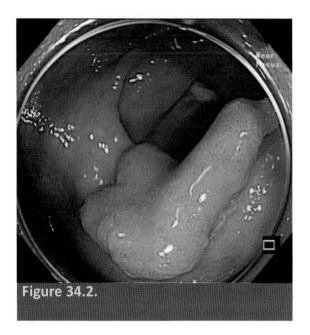

Figure 34.2.

Please describe what you see

A 20mm sessile lateral spreading tumour (non-granular type) is noted at the hepatic flexure.

In addition to white light endoscopic assessment, what further technique can be employed to characterise the lesion?

Image-enhanced endoscopic modalities, such as narrow band imaging (Figure 34.3).

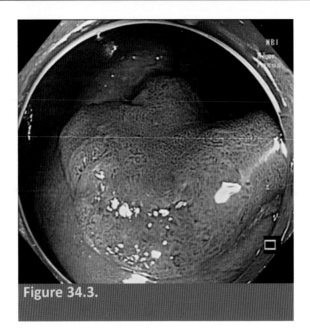

Figure 34.3.

Please describe what you see
A Kudo Type III vascular pattern on narrow band imaging.

What would you do next?

An endoscopic submucosal dissection (ESD).

An endoscopic submucosal resection is performed. Histology of the specimen reveals a tubular adenoma with low-grade dysplasia and the resection margin is clear.

Clinical pearls

- Screening of colorectal cancer should be offered to average-risk patients aged >50.
- Screening of colorectal cancer should be offered earlier if a patient has a positive family history of colorectal neoplasms.

- Image-enhanced endoscopy (IEE) techniques such as chromoendoscopy and narrow band imaging can be employed to characterise colorectal polyps.
- ESD is a safe and effective treatment for flat colorectal polyps.

Impress your attending

What is CEA? Would you recommend checking CEA in this patient?

CEA is carcinoembryonic antigen. It has a low sensitivity in the screening of colorectal cancer [8].

In patients who have been diagnosed with colorectal cancer, it could assist in staging and surgical planning. It is also the marker of choice for monitoring the response of metastatic disease to systemic therapy [9].

What is ESD? What are the common complications?

ESD involves mucosal resection along the middle to deep submucosal layer [10]. It offers *en bloc* resection of large colorectal polyps with a resection rate of around 90% [11].

Complications include:

- Infection.
- Bleeding.
- Perforation.
- Conversion to open surgery.

What are the rates of possible complications of colorectal ESD [12]?

- 2% bleeding risk.
- 2% perforation risk.

References

1. Rex D, Johnson D, Andersone J, *et al.* American College of Gastroenterology guidelines for colorectal cancer screening 2008. *Am J Gastroenterol* 2009; 104: 739-50.

2. Wong VWS, Wong GLH, Tsang SWC, *et al.* High prevalence of colorectal neoplasm in patients with non-alcoholic steatohepatitis. *Gut* 2011; 60(6): 829-36.

3. Ng SC, Lau JYW, Chan FKL, *et al.* Increased risk of advanced neoplasms among asymptomatic siblings of patients with colorectal cancer. *Gastroenterology* 2013; 144(3): 544-50.

4. Levin B, Lieberman DA, McFarland B, *et al.* Screening and surveillance for the early detection of colorectal cancer and adenomatous polyps, 2008: a joint guideline from the American Cancer Society, the US Multi-Society Task Force on Colorectal Cancer, and the American College of Radiology. *Gastroenterology* 2008; 134: 1570-95.

5. Lieberman DA. Screening for colorectal cancer. *N Engl J Med* 2009; 361(12): 1179-87.

6. Quintero E, Castells A, Bujandaet L, *et al.* Colonoscopy versus fecal immunochemical testing in colorectal-cancer screening. *N Engl J Med* 2012; 366(8): 697-706.

7. Lieberman DA, Harford WV, Ahnen DJ, *et al.* One-time screening for colorectal cancer with combined fecal occult-blood testing and examination of the distal colon. *N Engl J Med* 2001; 345: 555-60

8. Su B, Shi H, Wan J. Role of serum carcinoembryonic antigen in the detection of colorectal cancer before and after surgical resection. *World J Gastroenterol* 2012; 18(17): 2121-6.

9. Locker GY, Hamilton S, Harris J, *et al.* ASCO 2006 update of recommendations for the use of tumor markers in gastrointestinal cancer. *J Clin Oncol* 2006; 24: 5313-27.

10. Repici A, Pellicano R, Strangio G, *et al.* Endoscopic mucosal resection for early colorectal neoplasia: pathologic basis, procedures, and outcomes. *Dis Colon Rectum* 2009; 52: 1502-15.

11. Repici A, Hassan C, De Paula Pessoa D, *et al.* Efficacy and safety of endoscopic submucosal dissection for colorectal neoplasia: a systematic review. *Endoscopy* 2012; 44(02): 137-50.

12. ASGE Technology Committee; Maple JT, Abu Dayyeh BK, Chauhan SS, *et al.* Endoscopic submucosal dissection. *Gastrointest Endosc* 2015; 81(6): 1311-25.

Case 35

A 60-year-old gentleman with a history of osteoarthritis (OA) of the knee presents to the emergency department with tarry stools. He has no abdominal pain. He takes non-steroidal anti-inflammatory drugs (NSAIDs) intermittently for pain control.

Physical examination

- Temperature 37°C, pulse 120 bpm, BP 100/60mmHg, SaO_2 98-100% on RA.
- Hydration is satisfactory.
- Examination of the hands reveals no clubbing and normal-appearing palmar creases.
- Head and neck examination is unremarkable.
- Cardiovascular: HS dual, no murmur.
- His chest is clear on auscultation.
- Abdominal examination reveals a soft, non-tender abdomen.
- PR melaena.
- No signs of oedema.

Investigations

- CBC:
  - WBC 9 x 10^9/L;
  - haemoglobin 6.5g/dL;
  - platelets 330 x 10^9/L.
- Urea 20mmol/L.
- Creatinine 80μmol/L.
- Liver function tests are normal.

What is your differential diagnosis?

- Peptic ulcer bleeding (most likely).
- Upper GI neoplasm.
- Oesophageal or gastric varices — less likely as the patient does not have a history of chronic liver disease.
- Mallory-Weiss syndrome — less likely as the patient did not have preceding retching/vomiting.
- Angiodysplasia.
- Dieulafoy's lesion.

What further investigations would you order?

- Erect chest X-ray (CXR) (for free gas under the diaphragm to rule out perforation).

- Electrocardiogram (ECG).
- Oesophagogastroduodenoscopy (OGD).

CXR shows no free gas under the diaphragm. ECG shows a normal sinus rhythm.

An OGD is performed showing the pathology below (Figure 35.1).

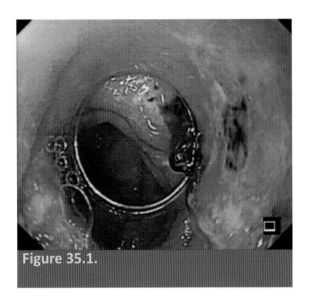

Figure 35.1.

Please describe what you see
This endoscopic image shows a distal D1/2 posterior wall ulcer with a visible vessel.

Adrenaline injection around the visible vessel followed by heater probe application is performed. The visible vessel is obliterated and the ulcer cavitated. A rapid urease test is negative.

What treatment should be given next?

An intravenous (IV) proton pump inhibitor (PPI) bolus, followed by a PPI infusion for 72 hours should be given to reduce the risk of rebleeding [1, 2].

Supportive transfusion is given. What is the target level of haemoglobin?

Hb ≥7g/dL in haemodynamically stable patients.

A restrictive transfusion strategy with transfusion given only when the haemoglobin level falls <7g/dL is associated with a better 6-week survival, less rebleeding and less complications [3].

On day-2 post-endoscopic therapy, the patient develops shock. Per rectal examination reveals fresh melaena. Fluid resuscitation and transfusion support are given.

What would you do next?

Repeat the OGD (Figure 35.2).

Most patients with recurrent bleeding can be successfully treated with repeat endoscopic therapy and avoid the need for surgery [4].

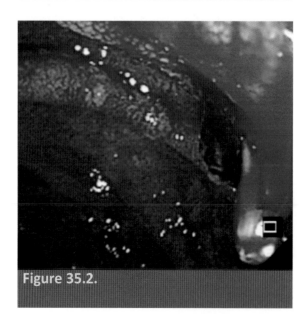

Figure 35.2.

Please describe what you see

The repeat OGD shows active oozing from a visible vessel at the posterior wall of the D1/2 junction which is the same lesion as the previous endoscopy. Endoscopic therapy with adrenaline injection and heater probe are applied. The ulcer is cavitated and haemostasis is achieved.

The patient remains stable after the second endoscopic therapy. He completes a course of IV PPI infusion. He passes yellow stools 3 days later. Haemoglobin remains stable and urea normalises.

A rapid urease test (RUT) was negative at the index endoscopy. Does the patient require additional testing for *Helicobacter pylori*?

Yes. Acute ulcer bleeding at the time of testing may decrease the sensitivity and negative predictive value of the RUT and hence further testing would be warranted after acute bleeding has settled [5, 6].

How would you advise the patient on the use of NSAIDs in the future?

This patient has a high gastrointestinal risk given his recent complicated peptic ulcer bleeding. He enjoyed good past health and his cardiovascular risk is considered low.

He should be advised against NSAIDs. If he must resume NSAIDs, daily PPI cover is indicated. Alternatively, a COX-2 inhibitor at the lowest effective dose plus daily PPI cover may offer the best protection against gastrointestinal side effects (Table 35.1) [7, 8].

Table 35.1. Recommendations for the prevention of complications due to NSAID-related ulcers.

<table>
<tr><td></td><td colspan="3">Gastrointestinal risk *</td></tr>
<tr><td></td><td>Low</td><td>Moderate</td><td>High</td></tr>
<tr><td>Low CV risk</td><td>NSAID alone (the least ulcerogenic NSAID at the lowest effective dose)</td><td>NSAID + PPI/misoprostol</td><td>Alternative therapy if possible or COX-2 inhibitor + PPI/ misoprostol</td></tr>
<tr><td>High CV risk** (low-dose aspirin required)</td><td>Naproxen + PPI/misoprostol</td><td>Naproxen + PPI/misoprostol</td><td>Avoid NSAIDs or COX-2 inhibitors Use alternative therapy</td></tr>
</table>

* Gastrointestinal risk is stratified into low (no risk factors), moderate (presence of one or two risk factors), and high (multiple risk factors, or previous ulcer complications, or concomitant use of corticosteroids or anticoagulants).

** High CV risk is arbitrarily defined as the requirement for low-dose aspirin for the prevention of serious CV events. All patients with a history of ulcers who require NSAIDs should be tested for *Helicobacter pylori*, and if the infection is present, eradication therapy should be given.

Clinical pearls

- A restrictive transfusion strategy should be employed in stable patients with ulcer bleeding.
- Repeat endoscopy is a reasonable option for patients who have had a first episode of ulcer rebleeding.
- An intravenous proton pump inhibitor infusion for 3 days should be given to patients who have a high risk of rebleeding.
- A rapid urease test may be inaccurate in the setting of active bleeding.

Impress your attending

What is the role of Hemospray® in the treatment of upper gastrointestinal bleeding?

Hemospray® is a nanopowder that promotes clotting which can be sprayed onto the bleeding site through upper endoscopy [9]. It may be used to treat Forrest Ia and Ib peptic ulcers. Haemostasis can be achieved in 95% of patients.

No major complications are reported.

References

1. Laine L, Jensen D. Management of patients with ulcer bleeding. *Am J Gastroenterol* 2012; 107: 345-60.
2. Laine L, McQuaid KR. Endoscopic therapy for bleeding ulcers: an evidence-based approach based on meta-analyses of randomized controlled trials. *Clin Gastroenterol Hepatol* 2009; 7: 33-47.
3. Villanueva C, Colomo A, Bosch A, *et al.* Transfusion strategies for acute upper gastrointestinal bleeding. *N Engl J Med* 2013; 368: 11-21.
4. Lau JY, Sung JJ, Lam YH, *et al.* Endoscopic retreatment compared with surgery in patients with recurrent bleeding after initial endoscopic control of bleeding ulcers. *N Engl J Med* 1999; 340: 751-6.
5. Chey WD, Wong BCY. Management of *Helicobacter pylori* infection. *Am J Gastroenterol* 2007; 102: 1808-25.
6. Lee JM, Breslin NP, Fallon C, *et al.* Rapid urease tests lack sensitivity in *Helicobacter pylori* diagnosis when peptic ulcer disease presents with bleeding. *Am J Gastroenterol* 2000; 95: 1166-70.
7. Chan FK, Wong VW, Suen BY, *et al.* Combination of a cyclo-oxygenase-2 inhibitor and a proton-pump inhibitor for prevention of recurrent ulcer bleeding in patients at very high risk: a double-blind, randomised trial. *Lancet* 2007; 369: 1621-6.
8. Lanza F, Chan FKL, Quigley E. Prevention of NSAID-related ulcer complications. *Am J Gastroenterol* 2009; 104: 728-38.

9. Sung JJ, Luo D, Wu JC, *et al.* Early clinical experience of the safety and effectiveness of Hemospray in achieving hemostasis in patients with acute peptic ulcer bleeding. *Endoscopy* 2011; 43(4): 291-5.

Case 36

History

A 58-year-old gentleman with a history of hypertension presents with a painless lump in the neck for 3 months. Fine needle aspiration of the mass and bone marrow examination shows a diffuse large B-cell lymphoma (DLBCL). Staging CT shows multiple enlarged lymph nodes in the neck, thorax and retroperitoneum (circles), compatible with stage IIIA DLBCL (Figures 36.1 to 36.3).

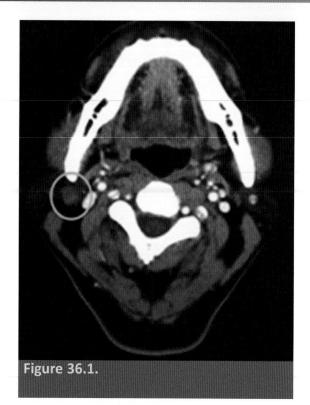

Figure 36.1.

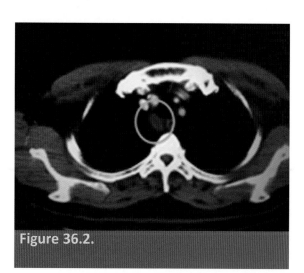

Figure 36.2.

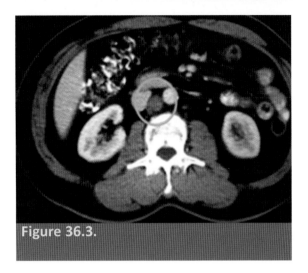

Figure 36.3.

Physical examination

- Temperature 37.2°C, pulse 72 bpm, BP 124/64mmHg, SaO_2 98-100% on RA.
- Alert, no flapping tremor.
- Examination of the hands reveals no clubbing and normal-appearing palmar creases.
- Head and neck examination is unremarkable with no lymph nodes palpable.
- Cardiovascular: HS dual, no murmur.
- His chest is clear on auscultation.
- Abdominal examination reveals a soft, non-tender abdomen, with no hepatosplenomegaly.
- No signs of oedema.

Investigations

- CBC:
  - WBC 9.6 x 10^9/L;
  - haemoglobin 12g/dL;
  - platelets 265 x 10^9/L.

- Bilirubin normal.
- ALP normal.
- ALT normal.

The patient is referred to an oncologist. A pre-chemotherapy work-up is done showing negative HBsAg, anti-HCV and anti-HIV. IgG anti-HBc is positive. HBV DNA is not checked.

Chemotherapy is commenced and the patient responds well to chemotherapy. A follow-up CT after the fifth cycle of treatment shows that most of the lymph nodes have resolved.

However, the patient develops jaundice before the sixth cycle of R-CHOP (rituximab, cyclophosphamide, hydroxydaunorubicin, Oncovin® and prednisolone). He is subsequently referred to the hepatology clinic for assessment.

What is the differential diagnosis?

- Flare up of hepatitis B.
- Other viral hepatitis (e.g. hepatitis A, E).
- Drug-induced liver injury.
- Budd-Chiari syndrome.
- Ischaemic hepatitis.

How would you assess the severity of the liver failure?

- History:
  - the presence of sleep-wake cycle disturbance;
  - the presence of jaundice.
- Physical examination:
  - Glasgow Coma Score;
  - the presence of a flapping tremor.

- Investigation:
  - bilirubin level;
  - clotting profile.

How would you perform the work-up for the cause of the liver failure?

- History:
  - the use of over-the-counter (OTC) medications or herbs;
  - abdominal pain.
- Physical examination:
  - tender hepatomegaly.
- Investigations:
  - viral markers: HBsAg, anti-HCV, HBV DNA level.

Apart from jaundice, the patient remains otherwise well. He has no sleep-wake cycle disturbance. He denies the use of OTC medications or herbal medicine. He has no abdominal pain.

Further examination shows no flapping tremor and no tender hepatomegaly.

Blood results are as follows:

- Bilirubin 616µmol/L.
- ALP 88 IU/L.
- ALT 1975 IU/L.
- INR 1.9.
- HBsAg positive, anti-HCV negative, HBV DNA 7 log IU/ml.

With the above information, what is the most likely cause of the liver failure?

Reactivation of occult hepatitis B.

What should be done next?

Stop chemotherapy (he was put on rituximab, cyclophosphamide, hydroxydaunorubicin, oncovin and prednisolone previously).

Commence antiviral therapy.

Chemotherapy is stopped and entecavir is started. The patient remains well and liver function is normalised 1 month later. HBV DNA becomes undetectable. Six months later, he is continued on entecavir. His DLBCL remains in remission and his HBV DNA levels are undetectable.

Clinical pearls

- In patients receiving immunosuppressants, hepatitis B reactivation is a potential hazard in both chronic hepatitis B and occult hepatitis B.
- Patients with chronic hepatitis B who are treated with immunosuppressants should receive antiviral prophylaxis.
- Patients with occult hepatitis B who are receiving immunosuppressants should have HBV DNA monitored. Antiviral prophylaxis should be given if HBV DNA is positive.

Impress your attending

What is the definition of occult hepatitis B?
Occult HBV infection is defined as the persistence of B virus genomes in HBsAg-negative individuals [1].

What is the risk of hepatitis B reactivation in patients with occult hepatitis B (HBsAg-negative, anti-HBc-positive) receiving rituximab?
Nearly 25% of occult hepatitis B patients who received rituximab without antiviral prophylaxis developed HBV reactivation [2].

What is the current recommendation of antiviral prophylaxis in patients receiving immunosuppressive therapy?

In the recently updated American Gastroenterological Association (AGA) guideline on the prevention and treatment of hepatitis B virus reactivation during immunosuppressive drug therapy, only patients at moderate to high risk undergoing immunosuppressive therapy should have antiviral prophylaxis [3].

Occult hepatitis B patients may have HBV DNA tested. Antiviral prophylaxis is recommended if HBV DNA is positive, otherwise, the HBV DNA level should be monitored [4, 5].

What is the preferred agent to be used?

Entecavir or tenofovir is recommended as studies have demonstrated reduced reactivation, hepatitis, mortality, and anticancer therapy interruption with these agents [4, 5].

How long should antiviral prophylaxis be continued for?

Antiviral therapy should be continued for at least 6-12 months after completion of immunosuppressant therapy (18 months for rituximab-based regimens according to the latest European Association for the Study of the Liver [EASL] clinical practice guidelines, 2017) [5].

References

1. Raimondo G, Allain JP, Brunetto MR, *et al.* Statements from the Taormina expert meeting on occult hepatitis B virus infection. *J Hepatol* 2008; 49: 652-7.
2. Yeo W, Chan TC, Leung NW, *et al.* Hepatitis B virus reactivation in lymphoma patients with prior resolved hepatitis B undergoing anticancer therapy with or without rituximab. *J Clin Oncol* 2009; 27: 605-11.
3. Reddy KR, Beavers KL, Hammond SP, *et al.* American Gastroenterological Association Institute guideline on the prevention and treatment of hepatitis B virus reactivation during

immunosuppressive drug therapy. *Gastroenterology* 2015; 148(1): 215-9.

4. https://www.aasld.org/sites/default/files/HBVGuidance_Terrault_et _al-2018-Hepatology.pdf.

5. http://www.easl.eu/medias/cpg/management-of-hepatitis-B-virus-infection/English-report.pdf.

Case 37

History

A 22-year-old gentleman with good past health presents to the outpatient clinic with a longstanding history of epigastric discomfort. He has no regurgitation. He has a normal appetite and has had no weight loss. He has no change of bowel habit, per-rectal bleeding, tarry stools and abdominal pain. He is not taking any medications or herbs.

Physical examination

- Temperature 37°C, pulse 72 bpm, BP 123/60mmHg, SaO_2 98-100% on RA.
- Hydration is satisfactory.
- Examination of the hands reveals no clubbing and normal-appearing palmar creases.
- Head and neck examination is unremarkable.
- Cardiovascular: HS dual, no murmur.
- His chest is clear on auscultation.
- Abdominal examination reveals a soft, non-tender abdomen.
- PR brown stool.
- No signs of oedema.

Investigations

- CBC:
  - WBC 9.3 x 10^9/L;
  - haemoglobin 12.3g/dL;
  - platelets 295 x 10^9/L.

What is your differential diagnosis of his epigastric discomfort?

- Peptic ulcer disease.
- Gastritis.
- Gastro-oesophageal reflux disease (GORD).
- Malignancy (e.g. liver, oesophageal, gastric).
- Pancreatic disease (chronic pancreatitis).
- Gastroparesis.
- Functional dyspepsia.

The patient is given an 8-week course of high-dose proton pump inhibitors (PPIs) but the symptoms persist.

What would be the next investigation?

Oesophagogastroduodenoscopy (OGD).

An OGD is performed which shows antral gastritis. An antral biopsy is taken (Figure 37.1).

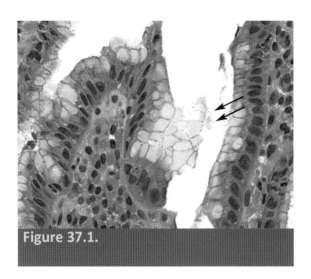

Figure 37.1.

Please describe what you see

The biopsy shows antral gastritis with the presence of *Helicobacter pylori* (arrows).

What are the different diagnostic tests for *Helicobacter pylori*?

Different diagnostic tests for *Helicobacter pylori* include the following [1]:

Invasive:

- Rapid urease test (RUT).
- Histology.
- Culture.
- Polymerase chain reaction.

Non-invasive:

- Urea breath test.
- Serology.
- Faecal antigen test.

What will affect the accuracy of a urea breath test?

PPI therapy can cause false-negative test results for 1-2 weeks [2, 3].

It is therefore suggested that PPIs should be withheld for 1-2 weeks before performing the RUT [1].

What would be your next step in the management of this patient?

H. pylori eradication therapy should be given.

What are the first-line regimens of *Helicobacter pylori* eradication?

The choice of first-line therapy should be based on the prevalence of clarithromycin resistance and local data on the efficacy of various treatment regimens.

In areas of low clarithromycin resistance (<15%), clarithromycin-containing treatments are recommended for first-line empirical treatment.

In areas of high clarithromycin resistance, bismuth-containing quadruple therapies are recommended for first-line empirical treatment. If this regimen is not available, a non-bismuth quadruple therapy is recommended.

What is the recommended dosing for a PPI in a *Helicobacter pylori* eradication regime?

Twice daily dosing of a proton pump inhibitor (PPI) in clarithromycin-based triple regimens is more effective than daily dosing [4].

What are the potential side effects of clarithromycin?

The patient should be warned about the side effects of clarithromycin, including GI upset, diarrhoea and altered taste [1].

Eradication is subsequently confirmed by a urea breath test.

Clinical pearls

- Twice daily dosing of a PPI in clarithromycin-based triple regimens is more effective than daily dosing.
- Confirmation of eradication should be done for all patients, preferably with a non-invasive test such as a urea breath test, unless a repeat endoscopy is required (thus gastric biopsies can be obtained).

Impress your attending

What are the possible ways to increase the efficacy of PPI-clarithromycin-containing triple therapies?

The use of high-dose, twice daily, more potent PPIs increases the efficacy of triple therapy.

Extending the duration of PPI-clarithromycin-containing triple therapies from 7 to 14 days improves the eradication success and should be considered [5].

What is sequential therapy?

Sequential therapy includes a 5-day period with a PPI and amoxicillin, followed by a 5-day period with a PPI, clarithromycin and metronidazole.

Sequential therapy may be more effective in patients with clarithromycin-resistant strains, as this regimen is postulated to select less resistant strains, and also cause destruction of the bacterial cell wall leading to a decrease in efflux pumps.

Side effects are similar with both treatment regimens and are rarely severe enough to cause discontinuation of therapy [6].

What is rifabutin? What is the potential role of rifabutin in Helicobacter pylori eradication?

Rifabutin is an antibiotic used in the treatment of tuberculosis.

It has been utilised as an alternative to clarithromycin in several small studies with eradication rates ranging from 38% to 91% [1].

What are the side effects of rifabutin?

Side effects of rifabutin include rash, gastrointestinal upset, deranged liver function tests and red discolouration of bodily fluids. Potentially serious side effects include myelotoxicity and ocular toxicity [1].

References

1. Chey WD, Wong BC; Practice Parameters Committee of the American College of Gastroenterology. American College of Gastroenterology guideline on the management of *Helicobacter pylori* infection. *Am J Gastroenterol* 2007; 102: 1808-25.
2. Chey WD, Woods M, Scheiman JM, *et al.* Lansoprazole and ranitidine affect the accuracy of the 14 C-urea breath test by a pH-dependent mechanism. *Am J Gastroenterol* 1997; 92: 446-50.
3. Laine L, Estrada R, Trujillo M, *et al.* Effect of proton-pump inhibitor therapy on diagnostic testing for *Helicobacter pylori*. *Ann Intern Med* 1998; 129: 547-50.

4. Vallve M, Vergara M, Gisbert JP, *et al.* Single vs. double dose of a proton pump inhibitor in triple therapy for *Helicobacter pylori* eradication: a meta-analysis. *Aliment Pharmacol Ther* 2002; 16: 1149-56.

5. Malfertheiner P, Megraud F, O'Morain CA, *et al*; European *Helicobacter* and Microbiota Study Group and Consensus Panel. Management of *Helicobacter pylori* infection - the Maastricht V/Florence Consensus Report. *Gut* 2017; 66(1): 6-30.

6. Vaira D, Zullo A, Vakil N, *et al.* Sequential therapy versus standard triple-drug therapy for *Helicobacter pylori* eradication: a randomized trial. *Ann Intern Med* 2007; 146: 556-63.

Case 38

A 53-year-old gentleman with good past health presents to the outpatient clinic with a 3-month history of malaise and shortness of breath on exertion. He has a normal appetite and no weight loss.

Physical examination

- Temperature 37°C, pulse 120 bpm, BP 100/60mmHg, SaO$_2$ 98-100% on RA.
- Hydration is satisfactory.
- Examination of the hands reveals no clubbing and normal-appearing palmar creases.
- Head and neck examination is unremarkable.
- Cardiovascular: HS dual, no murmur.
- His chest is clear on auscultation.
- Abdominal examination reveals a soft, non-tender abdomen.
- PR melaena.
- No signs of oedema.

Investigations

- CBC:
  - WBC 9.6 x 10^9/L;
  - haemoglobin 6g/dL;
  - platelets 265 x 10^9/L.
- Pre-transfusion blood results:
  - MCV 74fL;
  - serum iron 5μmol/L;
  - TIBC 80μmol/L;
  - ferritin 25pmol/L;
  - blood film shows hypochromic red blood cells with poikilocytosis and anisocytosis.
- Post-transfusion haemoglobin level is 9.5g/dL.

What is the differential diagnosis of microcytic anaemia [1]?

- Iron deficiency anaemia.
- Thalassaemia.
- Anaemia of chronic illness.
- Sideroblastic anaemia.

What are the typical features of the CBC and iron profile for the possible causes of microcytic anaemia?

The typical features of the CBC and iron profile for the possible causes of microcytic anaemia are listed in Table 38.1.

Table 38.1. Differential diagnosis of microcytic anaemia [1].				
	Iron deficiency	**Anaemia of chronic illness**	**Thalassaemia trait**	**Sideroblastic anaemia**
MCV	↓	↓ or normal	↓↓↓	↓
Serum iron	↓	↓	Normal	↑
Serum TIBC	↑	↓	Normal	Normal
Serum ferritin	↓	Normal or ↑	Normal	↑

With the above results, what is the most likely cause of microcytic anaemia in this patient?

Iron deficiency anaemia.

What would be the next investigation?

Oesophagogastroduodenoscopy (OGD).

An OGD is performed which shows a clean stomach with normal mucosa down to D2.

What should be done next?

A colonoscopy.

A colonoscopy is performed with good bowel preparation and complete colonic examination. The terminal ileum is intubated and is normal up to 20cm from the ileocecal valve. Two colonic polyps sized 3mm are removed from the rectum. No blood is seen.

What would you do next?

Capsule endoscopy (CE).

In patients with suspected occult obscure GI bleeding (OGIB), in the absence of localising signs or symptoms, small-bowel evaluation is recommended after an initial negative OGD and colonoscopy [2].

CE is recommended as the first-line diagnostic tool for evaluation of the small bowel in patients with OGIB [2].

Capsule endoscopy is performed and the pathology is shown in Figure 38.1.

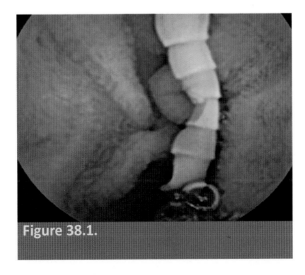

Figure 38.1.

Please describe what you see

The capsule endoscopy image reveals a tapeworm.

What is the treatment for tapeworm infection [3]?

Treatment is one of the following:

- Albendazole 15mg/kg daily for 8 days.
- Praziquantel 50mg/kg daily for 10 days.

The patient is given albenazole for 8 days according to the protocol. He is currently stable with a haemoglobin level of 12g/dL.

Clinical pearls

- An iron profile should be ordered to confirm iron deficiency in patients with microcytic anaemia.
- Capsule endoscopy is the investigation of choice for patients with suspected occult obscure GI bleeding after a negative OGD and colonoscopy.
- Praziquantel and albendazole are the treatment choices for tapeworm infection.

Impress your attending

What are the common capsule endoscopic findings in patients with unexplained iron deficiency anaemia after a negative OGD and colonoscopy [4]?

- Positive findings are noted in 57% of patients.
- Angiodysplasias (24%).
- Multiple jejunal or ileal ulcers (12%).
- Multiple erosions (8%).
- Tumours (4%).

- Ulcers (6%).
- Polyps (4%).

What are the different types of tapeworm infection [5]?
- *Taenia saginata* (beef tapeworm).
- *Taenia solium* (pork tapeworm).
- *Taenia asiatica* (pork tapeworm).

What is the epidemiology of tapeworm [5]?
- *Taenia saginata* and *Taenia solium* are worldwide in distribution.
- *Taenia asiatica* is limited to Asia and is seen mostly in the Republic of Korea, China, Taiwan, Indonesia and Thailand.

What do you know about the life cycle of tapeworms [5]?
- Humans are the definitive host.
- Eggs or gravid proglottids are passed with faeces and infect the intermediate host — cattle (*T. saginata*) and pigs (*T. solium* and *T. asiatica*).
- Humans become infected by ingesting raw or undercooked infected meat.
- In the human intestine, the cysticercus develops over 2 months into an adult tapeworm and resides in the small intestine.
- The adult tapeworm produces proglottids which mature, become gravid, detach from the tapeworm, and migrate to the anus or are passed in the stool (approximately 6 per day).

References

1. Kumar and Clark. *Clinical Medicine*, 5th ed. London, UK: Saunders, 2011: 415.
2. The role of endoscopy in the management of obscure GI bleeding. *Gastrointest Endosc* 2010; 72: 471-9.
3. Kumar and Clark. *Clinical Medicine*, 5th ed. London, UK: Saunders, 2011: 119.

4. Apostolopoulos P, Liatsos C, Gralnek IM, *et al.* The role of wireless capsule endoscopy in investigating unexplained iron deficiency anaemia after negative endoscopic evaluation of the upper and lower gastrointestinal tract. *Endoscopy* 2006; 38: 1127-32.

5. http://www.cdc.gov/dpdx/taeniasis/index.html.

Case 39

A 20-year-old lady presents with frequent urination. She has no abdominal pain, pruritis, fever or jaundice. There is no family history of diabetes.

Physical examination

- Temperature 36.7°C, pulse 66 bpm, BP 100/53mmHg, SaO_2 98-100% on RA.
- Alert, no jaundice, no stigmata of chronic liver disease.
- Examination of the hands reveals no clubbing and normal-appearing palmar creases.
- Head and neck examination is unremarkable, with no lymph nodes palpable.
- Cardiovascular: HS dual, no murmur.
- Her chest is clear on auscultation.
- Abdominal examination reveals a soft, non-tender abdomen, with no organomegaly.
- No signs of oedema.

Investigations

- CBC is normal.
- Bilirubin 12µmol/L.
- ALP 1375 IU/L (incidental finding).
- ALT 115 IU/L (incidental finding).
- Renal function is normal.

What is your differential diagnosis?

- Biliary obstruction.
- Hepatocellular disease, e.g. cirrhosis, alcoholic liver disease.
- Drug-induced cholestasis.
- Hepatocellular carcinoma.
- Infiltrative disease, e.g. tuberculosis, sarcoidosis.
- Primary biliary cirrhosis (PBC).
- Primary sclerosing cholangitis (PSC).

What further history would you enquire?

- Drinking history.
- Drug history including herbs and over-the-counter medications.

She drinks 3-4 cans of beer per day. She is not taking any regular medications but she admits to using recreational drugs including ketamine.

What further blood tests would you order for the work-up of the underlying aetiology of deranged liver function?

* Anti-mitochondria antibody (AMA).
* HIV status.

AMA and HIV are negative.

What other tests would you order?

Ultrasound (USG) of the abdomen.

USG of the abdomen shows irregular fatty infiltration of the liver; otherwise there are no biliary stones or biliary dilatation. There is right hydronephrosis.

A liver biopsy is performed (Figures 39.1 to 39.3).

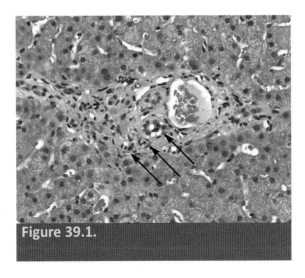

Figure 39.1.

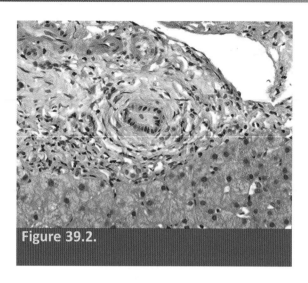

Figure 39.2.

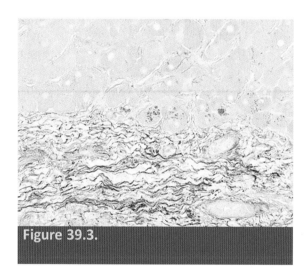

Figure 39.3.

Please describe what you see

Interlobular bile ducts are present and show focal epithelial disarray and an intraepithelial lymphocytic infiltrate.

There is a mild ductular reaction and chronic cholestasis, which is featured by deposition of copper-associated protein in periportal hepatocytes.

There are no features suggestive of primary biliary cirrhosis or primary sclerosing cholangitis.

What is the most likely unifying diagnosis?

Ketamine-induced liver and bladder injury.

The patient stops using ketamine and her liver function gradually improves.

Clinical pearls

- One in ten ketamine abusers suffer from liver injury.
- Ketamine may affect the liver by parenchymal injury and affecting smooth muscle of the sphincter of Oddi that leads to large bile duct dilatation.
- Sustained abstinence from ketamine abuse is protective against liver injury.

Impress your attending

What is ketamine?
Ketamine is a dissociative anaesthetic agent. It may be misused as a recreational hallucinogenic drug [1].

What are the effects of ketamine?
It gives excitement, dream-like states, hallucinations and vivid imagery [2].

What is the mechanism of biliary injury by ketamine?
Ketamine may affect the liver in two different ways: parenchymal injury with bile ductular damage and affecting smooth muscle of the sphincter of Oddi that leads to large bile duct dilatation [3].

What is the prevalence of liver dysfunction in ketamine abusers [3]?
It is reported that liver injury is encountered in one-tenth of patients.

What other potential damage is caused by ketamine misuse [4]?

- Cardiovascular: arrhythmias, bradycardia or tachycardia, hypertension or hypotension.
- Gastrointestinal: anorexia, nausea, increased salivation, vomiting.
- Neuromuscular and skeletal: increased skeletal muscle tone (tonic-clonic movements).
- Ocular: diplopia, increased intraocular pressure, nystagmus.
- Respiratory: airway obstruction, apnoea, increased bronchial secretions, respiratory depression, laryngospasm.
- Renal: hydronephrosis, ketamine-induced ulcerative cystitis and renal papillary necrosis [5].

References

1. Lo RS, Krishnamoorthy R, Freeman JG, Austin AS. Cholestasis and biliary dilatation associated with chronic ketamine abuse: a case series. *Singapore Med J* 2011; 52(3): e52-5.
2. Gutkin E, Hussain SA, Sang HK. Ketamine-induced biliary dilatation: from Hong Kong to New York. *J Addict Med* 2012; 6(1): 89-91.
3. Wong GL-H, Tam YH, Ng CF, *et al.* Liver injury is common among chronic abusers of ketamine. *Clin Gastroenterol Hepatol* 2014; 12(10): 1759-62.
4. Ketamine. Merck Manual. Drug information provided by Lexi-Comp, May 2014.
5. Middela S, Pearce I. Ketamine-induced vesicopathy: a literature review. *Int J Clin Practice* 2011; 65(1): 27-30.

Case 40

History

A 34-year-old gentleman with good past health presents to the emergency department with on and off rectal bleeding for 2 weeks. He has had no vomiting or haematemesis. He has no abdominal pain, fever or anaemic symptoms. He denies the use of pain killers and he is not on aspirin.

Physical examination

- Temperature 37°C, pulse 80 bpm, BP 123/63mmHg, SaO_2 98-100% on RA.
- Hydration satisfactory.
- Examination of the hands reveals no clubbing and normal-appearing palmar creases.
- Head and neck examination is unremarkable.
- Cardiovascular: HS dual, no murmur.
- His chest is clear on auscultation.
- Abdominal examination reveals a soft, non-tender abdomen.
- PR old blood.
- No signs of oedema.

Investigations

- CBC:
  - WBC 8 x 10^9/L;
  - haemoglobin 7.2g/dL;
  - platelets 234 x 10^9/L.
- Urea 3.4mmol/L.
- Creatinine 80µmol/L.

What is the differential diagnosis of per rectal bleeding?

- Diverticular bleeding.
- Ischaemic colitis.
- Infectious colitis.
- Vascular ectasia.
- Haemorrhoids.
- Carcinoma.
- Inflammatory bowel disease.
- Colonic ulcers.
- Radiation proctitis.
- Meckel's diverticulum.

What is the next investigation?

Oesophagogastroduodenoscopy (OGD).

An OGD is performed and shows a clean stomach with normal mucosa down to D2.

What should be done next?

A colonoscopy.

A colonoscopy is performed with good bowel preparation and complete colonic examination. The terminal ileum is intubated and is normal up to 20cm from the ileocecal valve. Some old blood is seen passing from above.

In view of the patient's young age with overt obscure GI bleeding, it raises the suspicion of a Meckel's diverticulum. A 99mTc-pertechnetate Meckel's scan is arranged but it shows a normal result.

What is the sensitivity of a 99mTc-pertechnetate Meckel's scan?

A 99mTc-pertechnetate Meckel's scan has the best results when used in children with a sensitivity of 80-90% and a specificity of 95% [1]. However, when applied to adults, the sensitivity drops to 62% and a specificity of 9% [2, 3].

A computed tomography enteroclysis is also arranged (Figure 40.1).

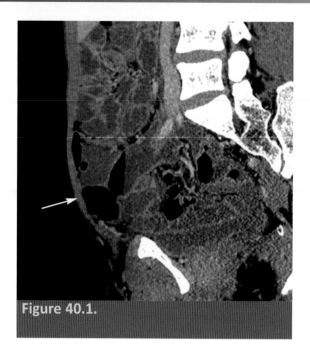

Figure 40.1.

Please describe what you see

This oblique coronal reformatted image shows an air-filled blind-ending pouch (arrow) arising from the antimesenteric border of the distal ileum (arrowheads).

What is your diagnosis?

Meckel's diverticulum.

The patient is referred to the surgical team for resection of the Meckel's diverticulum. The surgery is uneventful and he has no recurrence of gastrointestinal bleeding.

Clinical pearls

- Meckel's diverticulum is a possible cause of GI bleeding of obscure origin.
- A 99mTc-pertechnetate Meckel's scan is best used in children. The sensitivity and specificity of a Meckel's scan decreases in adults.

Impress your attending

What is a Meckel's diverticulum?

It is the most common congenital anomaly of the gastrointestinal tract and arises from the incomplete obliteration of the omphalomesenteric duct in the 7th week of gestation [4]. This leads to a true diverticulum (with the presence of all layers of the small bowel wall) developing from the anti-mesenteric surface of the mid-distal ileum.

What is the 'rule of two' in Meckel's diverticulum [5]?

The 'rule of two' exemplifies the classical presentation of Meckel's diverticulum:

- Located 2 feet proximal to the ileocecal valve.
- Presents before the age of 2 years.
- Seen twice as commonly in men as women.
- Found in ~2% of the population.

What is the complication rate and the most common complication of a Meckel's diverticulum?

Only 2-4% patients will develop a Meckel's diverticulum-related complication during their lifetimes [6].

Gastrointestinal bleeding is the most common manifestation in adults [6].

In the presence of ectopic tissue, e.g. gastric and pancreatic tissues [5], it leads to acid secretion and consequently to mucosal ulceration downstream from the diverticulum.

Hence, an obscure or overt GI bleeding may rarely occur in patients with a Meckel's diverticulum.

What are the causes of false-positive and false-negative results of 99mTc-pertechnetate Meckel's scans in patients with a Meckel's diverticulum?

False positives have been known to arise from other sites that contain ectopic gastric mucosa, as well as from vascular anomalies, bowel ulceration, inflammation and obstruction.

False negatives occur when the ectopic gastric tissue in the diverticulum is very minimal or when the scintigraphic activity is diluted due to a sudden haemorrhage or bowel hypersecretion [5].

References

1. Jewett TC Jr, Duszynski DO, Allen JE. The visualization of Meckel's diverticulum with 99mTc-pertechnetate. *Surgery* 1970; 68: 567-70.
2. Lin S, Suhocki PV, Ludwig KA, Shetzline MA. Gastrointestinal bleeding in adult patients with Meckel's diverticulum: the role of technetium 99m pertechnetate scan. *South Med J* 2002; 95: 1338-41.
3. Sagar J, Kumar V, Shah DK. Meckel's diverticulum: a systematic review. *J R Soc Med* 2006; 99: 501-5.
4. Chan KW. Perforation of Meckel's diverticulum caused by a chicken bone: a case report. *J Med Case Reports* 2009; 3: 48.
5. Uppal K, Tubbs RS, Matusz P, *et al.* Meckel's diverticulum: a review. *Clin Anat* 2011; 24(4): 416-22.
6. Fernandes C, Pinho R, Carvalho J. Meckel's diverticulum: a rare cause of overt obscure gastrointestinal bleeding in an adult male. *GE Port J Gastroenterol* 2015; 22(3): 121-2.

Case 41

A 29-year-old gentleman with a history of extensive ulcerative colitis (UC) returns for a clinic follow-up. His disease is well controlled. He has no fever or abdominal pain.

Physical examination

- Temperature 36.8°C, pulse 72 bpm, BP 110/72mmHg, SaO_2 98-100% on RA.
- Alert, no jaundice with no stigmata of chronic liver disease.
- Examination of the hands reveals no clubbing and normal-appearing palmar creases.
- Head and neck examination is unremarkable, with no lymph nodes palpable.
- Cardiovascular: HS dual. No murmur.
- His chest is clear on auscultation.
- Abdominal examination reveals a soft, non-tender abdomen, with no organomegaly.
- No signs of oedema.

Investigations

- CBC:
  - WBC 9.7 x 10^9/L;
  - haemoglobin 10g/dL;
  - platelets 265 x 10^9/L.
- Bilirubin 15μmol/L.
- ALP 350 IU/L.
- ALT 50 IU/L (baseline normal).
- Renal function is normal.

What are the common causes of increased ALP?

- Physiological.
- Adolescence.
- Pregnancy.
- Pathological.
- Bile obstruction.
- Hepatocellular disease, e.g. cirrhosis, hepatitis, alcoholic liver disease.

- Drug-induced.
- Hepatocellular carcinoma.
- Infiltrative disease, e.g. TB, sarcoidosis.
- Primary biliary cirrhosis.
- Primary sclerosing cholangitis (PSC).
- Bone disease.

How would you evaluate the origin of ALP?

- ALP isoenzyme.
- Gamma-glutamyltransferase (GGT).

The GGT level is elevated. A CT scan with contrast is performed as shown below (Figures 41.1 [arterial phase] and 41.2 [portal venous phase]).

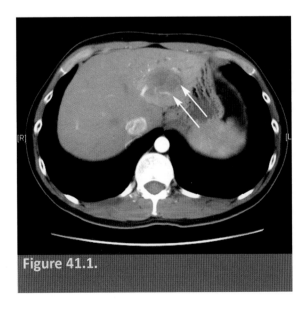

Figure 41.1.

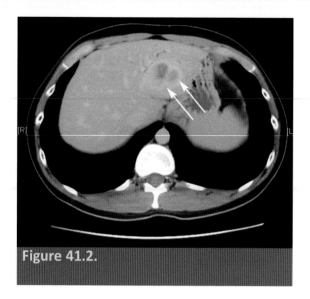

Figure 41.2.

Please describe what you see

A large mass is present in the left lobe of the liver (arrows). It is hypoenhancing on the arterial phase and shows progressive internal enhancement on the portal venous and delayed phases. The liver appears non-cirrhotic. The intrahepatic ducts in the left lobe are mildly dilated.

What is the most likely diagnosis, given the background of the patient?

- Cholangiocarcinoma on a background of PSC.
- Hepatocellular carcinoma is less likely given the lack of risk factors and a non-cirrhotic liver.

A further work-up shows no evidence of distant metastasis. A robotic left hepatectomy is performed.

Histology shows a poorly differentiated intrahepatic cholangiocarcinoma on a background of sclerosing cholangitis with periportal fibrosis, consistent with primary sclerosing cholangitis.

In addition to cholangiocarcinoma, what are the other cancers that the patient is at risk of?

- Colorectal cancer [1].
- Gallbladder cancer [2].

The patient is offered an annual colonoscopy with chromoendoscopy for screening of colorectal cancer. Annual ultrasound is also offered for screening of recurrence of cholangiocarcinoma and for gallbladder cancer. His underlying ulcerative colitis is well controlled by mesalazine.

Clinical pearls

- PSC is associated with IBD.
- PSC is a risk factor for malignancy, namely colorectal carcinoma, cholangiocarcinoma and gallbladder cancer. Regular surveillance is warranted to mitigate the risks of developing these neoplasms.
- Medical treatment options are limited for PSC.

Impress your attending

What is the association of PSC with IBD [3]?
- There is a strong association of IBD with PSC.
- The prevalence of IBD in PSC is 60%-80%.
- However, IBD may be diagnosed at any time during the course of PSC. In the majority of cases, the diagnosis of IBD precedes that of PSC, some concomitantly, and some where IBD is diagnosed after PSC.

What are the characteristics of IBD in patients with PSC [3]?
- Extensive colitis.
- More indolent/mild disease.
- More fluctuating course.
- Rectal-sparing.
- Backwash ileitis.

- Higher risk of colorectal neoplasms.
- Higher risk of pouchitis.

What is the role of ursodeoxycholic acid in the treatment of PSC?

Some data suggest that ursodeoxycholic acid improves abnormal liver function tests, but not the histology and prognosis in PSC, while high-dose ursodeoxycholic acid may be harmful [4, 5]. Therefore, current guidelines recommend against the use of ursodeoxycholic acid in the treatment of PSC [3].

References

1. Broome U, Bergquist A. Primary sclerosing cholangitis, inflammatory bowel disease, and colon cancer. *Semin Liver Dis* 2006; 26: 31-41.
2. Said K, Glaumann H, Bergquist A. Gallbladder disease in patients with primary sclerosing cholangitis. *J Hepatol* 2008; 48: 598-605.
3. Chapman R, Fevery J, Kalloo A, *et al.* Diagnosis and management of primary sclerosing cholangitis. *Hepatol* 2010; 51: 660-78.
4. Van Assche G, Dignass A, Reinisch W, *et al*; European Crohn's and Colitis Organisation (ECCO). The second European evidence-based Consensus on the diagnosis and management of Crohn's disease: special situations. *J Crohn's Colitis* 2010; 4(1): 63-101.
5. Lindor KD, Kowdley KV, Luketic VA, *et al.* High-dose ursodeoxycholic acid for the treatment of primary sclerosing cholangitis. *Hepatol* 2009; 50: 808-14.

Case 42

History

A 54-year-old lady presents with biliary pancreatitis complicated with respiratory failure requiring intensive care admission. She subsequently reports an increase in abdominal distension and persistent abdominal discomfort. She has no fever or jaundice. She is a non-drinker. She has a past history of hypertension. She is taking lisinopril and denies over-the-counter medications. She has been scheduled for a cholecystectomy.

Physical examination

- Temperature 37.5°C, pulse 72 bpm, BP 124/72mmHg, SaO_2 98-100% on RA.
- Hydration satisfactory.
- Examination of the hands reveals no clubbing and normal-appearing palmar creases.
- Head and neck examination is unremarkable.
- Cardiovascular: HS dual, no murmur.
- Auscultation of her chest reveals right lower zone crepitation.
- Abdominal examination reveals a soft abdomen, with mild epigastric tenderness, no peritoneal signs, a vague epigastric mass and no detectable ascites.
- No signs of oedema.

Investigations

- CBC:
  - WBC 8×10^9/L;
  - haemoglobin 12.2g/dL;
  - platelets 285×10^9/L.
- Total bilirubin 22μmol/L.
- ALP 32 IU/L.
- ALT 22 IU/L.
- Albumin 38g/L.
- Creatinine 80μmol/L.
- INR 1.1.
- Amylase normal.

What is your differential diagnosis specific to her situation?

Given her recent history of biliary pancreatitis, the following differential diagnoses should be considered:

- Pancreatic pseudocyst formation.

- Recurrent pancreatitis.
- Pancreatic ascites.

What other tests would you request?

Imaging of the pancreas (contrast CT or endoscopic ultrasound).

A contrast CT of the abdomen is arranged (Figure 42.1).

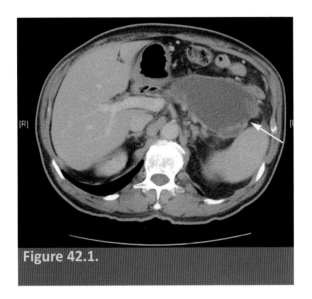

Figure 42.1.

Please describe what you see
A unilocular fluid collection with a thin, well-defined enhancing wall is present at the pancreatic body and tail (arrow).

What is the diagnosis?

Given the history of preceding pancreatitis and classical CT appearance, the diagnosis is a pancreatic pseudocyst.

What is a pseudocyst?

It is a localised fluid collection that lacks an epithelial lining; rather the cyst wall consists of inflammatory and fibrous tissue.

What is the risk of pancreatic fluid collection progressing into the formation of pseudocysts after an episode of pancreatitis?

Approximately half of pancreatic fluid collections will resolve within 6 weeks, and up to 15% will persist as encapsulated pseudocysts [1].

Which type of pseudocyst can be managed conservatively?

Pseudocysts which are small (<6cm) and asymptomatic may be managed conservatively [2].

What are the possible complications of a pseudocyst [2]?

- Abdominal pain.
- Obstruction to surrounding organs (duodenum, stomach or bile duct).
- Infection.
- Rupture.
- Bleeding.

In view of the large size of the pseudocyst and the complication (abdominal pain), drainage of the cyst is warranted. What are the possible ways of drainage?

Drainage of the pseudocyst can be done surgically, radiologically or endoscopically [2].

EUS-guided drainage of the pseudocyst is successfully performed. The abdominal distension and abdominal pain resolves after the drainage.

Clinical pearls

- Pancreatic pseudocyst is a complication of pancreatitis.
- Pancreatic pseudocyst may be managed conservatively if it is small (<6cm) and asymptomatic.
- Drainage of the pseudocyst can be done surgically, radiologically or endoscopically.

Impress your attending

What is the efficacy of endoscopic as compared with surgical cystogastrostomy?
Endoscopic drainage is comparable to surgical cystogastrostomy for pancreatic pseudocyst drainage [3].

Endoscopic treatment is associated with shorter hospital stays, less morbidity and lower cost [3].

Is antibiotic prophylaxis needed before EUS-guided pseudocyst drainage?
Yes, antibiotic prophylaxis is recommended according to the latest American Society for Gastrointestinal Endoscopy (ASGE) guideline [4].

Fluoroquinolone may be considered as the antibiotic of choice [4].

References

1. Baillie J. Pancreatic pseudocysts (part I). *Gastrointest Endosc* 2004; 59: 873-9.
2. DiMagno EP, Reber HA, Tempero MA. AGA technical review on the epidemiology, diagnosis, and treatment of pancreatic ductal adenocarcinoma. *Gastroenterology* 1999; 117(6): 1464-84.

3.   Varadarajulu S, Bang JY, Sutton BS, *et al.* Equal efficacy of endoscopic and surgical cystogastrostomy for pancreatic pseudocyst drainage in a randomized trial. *Gastroenterology* 2013; 145(3): 583-90.

4.   ASGE Standards of Practice Committee; Banerjee S, Shen B, Baron TH, *et al.* Antibiotic prophylaxis for GI endoscopy. *Gastrointest Endosc* 2008; 67: 791-8.

Case 43

A 63-year-old lady with a history of lymphoma complicated with cord compression presents to the surgical department with generalised abdominal discomfort and distension. She has no fever, jaundice or gastrointestinal bleeding symptoms. There are no urinary symptoms. She is bedbound due to lower limb weakness secondary to the cord compression.

Physical examination

- Temperature 37.2°C, pulse 64 bpm, BP 103/62mmHg, SaO_2 98-100% on RA.
- Hydration satisfactory.
- Examination of the hands reveals no clubbing and normal-appearing palmar creases.
- Head and neck examination is unremarkable.
- Cardiovascular: HS dual, no murmur.
- Auscultation of her chest reveals right lower zone crepitation.
- Abdominal examination reveals a soft, non-tender abdomen, with mild distension and no shifting dullness.
- No signs of oedema.

Investigations

- CBC:
  - WBC 4.5 x 10^9/L;
  - haemoglobin 9.2g/dL;
  - platelets 295 x 10^9/L.
- Total bilirubin 9µmol/L.
- ALP 65 IU/L.
- ALT 22 IU/L.
- Albumin 30g/L.
- Creatinine 45µmol/L.
- INR 1.05.
- Serum potassium normal.
- Adjusted calcium normal.
- Amylase level normal.
- Thyroid function test is normal.

What are the possible causes of generalised abdominal distension?

The causes of generalised abdominal distension can be memorised using the mnemonic "6Fs":

- Fat (obesity).
- Faeces (constipation).
- Fetus (pregnancy).
- Flatus (gaseous distension).
- Fluid (ascites).
- Fatal growth (neoplasm).

What are the organic causes of constipation [1]?

- Drugs:
  - opiates;
  - calcium channel blockers;
  - anti-Parkinson medications;
  - aluminium;
  - calcium;
  - iron supplements;
  - anticholinergics;
  - antispasmotics;
  - vincristine.
- Mechanical obstruction:
  - colorectal cancer;
  - external compression;
  - anal fissure.
- Metabolic conditions:
  - hypothyroidism;
  - hypercalcaemia;
  - hypokalaemia;
  - diabetes mellitus;
  - heavy metal poisoning;

- myopathies;
- amyloidosis;
- scleroderma.
- Neuropathy:
  - Parkinson's disease;
  - spinal cord injury;
  - Chagas disease.
- Others:
  - depression;
  - immobility.

A contrast CT of the abdomen is arranged by the surgical team (Figure 43.1).

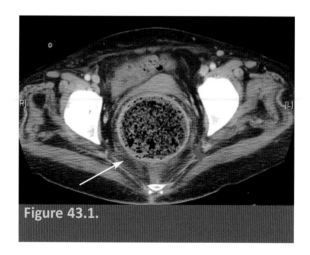

Figure 43.1.

Please describe what you see

The rectum is markedly distended (arrow) and impacted with faecal material.

The rectal wall is mildly thickened and is associated with inflammatory stranding and a small amount of fluid (arrowhead) in the perirectal fat suggestive of proctitis.

On further questioning, the patient has had longstanding constipation.

Given the history and the imaging findings, what is the diagnosis?

Given the history of this patient's bedbound state, longstanding constipation and a grossly distended faecal-loaded rectum associated with proctitis, the most likely diagnosis is stercoral proctitis.

What is the management?

Conservative treatment with laxatives and a periodic enema should be considered as the first line of treatment [1, 2].

Approximately 40% of patients with megarectum and megacolon referred for surgery respond to conservative treatment [3].

Patients not responsive to conservative treatment may be treated successfully by surgery [3]. A proctectomy and coloanal anastomosis, restorative proctocolectomy, and panproctocolectomy with a defunctioning stoma are all possible surgical options.

Clinical pearls

- Chronic constipation may lead to dilated bowels.
- A grossly distended bowel may lead to bowel ischaemia, inflammation and even perforation.
- Conservative treatment with laxatives and a periodic enema is the first-line treatment of stercoral proctitis.
- Patients failing conservative treatment may be treated by surgery.

Impress your attending

What is the pathophysiology of stercoral proctitis?

With a grossly distended intestine, the bowel wall is stretched thin, with the blood supply to the affected area decreasing as the intraluminal pressure increases. Ischaemic pressure can lead to proctitis.

Severe cases may be complicated with necrosis and ulceration, rectal bleeding, focal thickening of the colonic wall and even perforation [4-6].

References

1. Bharucha AE, Pemberton JH, Locke III GR. American Gastroenterological Association technical review on constipation. *Gastroenterology* 2013; 144(1): 218.
2. Silva M, Cardoso H, Macedo G. A severe case of bowel impaction. *Int J Colorectal Dis* 2016: 31(4): 917-8.
3. Suilleabhain CBO, Anderson JH, McKee RF, Finlay IG. Strategy for the surgical management of patients with idiopathic megarectum and megacolon. *Br J Surg* 2001; 88: 1392-6.
4. Heffernan C, Pachter HL, Megibow AJ, *et al*. Stercoral colitis leading to fatal peritonitis: CT findings. *AJR Am J Roentgenol* 2005; 184: 1189-93.
5. Haddad R, Bursle G, Piper B. Stercoral perforation of the sigmoid colon. *Aus N Z J Surg* 2005; 75: 244-6.
6. Dubinsky I. Stercoral perforation of the colon: case report and review of the literature. *J Emerg Med* 1996; 14: 323-5.

Case 44

A 54-year-old Chinese gentleman presents with a 2-week history of right-sided abdominal pain, abdominal distension, haemoptysis and fever. Physical exam shows a distended abdomen and a Ryle's tube is inserted, with high output noted. He is also started on broad-spectrum antibiotics.

Physical examination

- Afebrile, pulse 80 bpm, BP 120/80mmHg, SaO_2 98-100% on RA.
- Hydration is satisfactory.
- Examination of the hands reveals no clubbing and normal-appearing palmar creases.
- Head and neck examination is unremarkable.
- Cardiovascular: HS dual, no murmur.
- His chest is clear on auscultation.
- Abdominal examination reveals a soft, non-tender abdomen, with no peritoneal signs.
- No signs of oedema.

Investigations

- CBC:
  - WBC 9.6 x 10^9/L (raised eosinophil differential of 31%);
  - haemoglobin 9.8g/dL;
  - platelets 825 x 10^9/L.
- CRP 237mg/L.
- Blood culture: *Klebsiella*.
- Albumin 28g/L.
- Liver function tests are normal.
- Creatinine 60μmol/L.

What further investigations would you request?

In view of his abdominal symptoms, computed tomography (CT) scans of the thorax, abdomen and pelvis are performed (Figures 44.1 and 44.2).

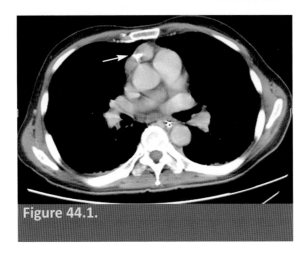

Figure 44.1.

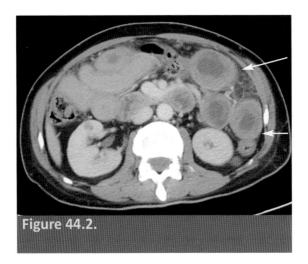

Figure 44.2.

Please describe what you see

Figure 44.1 is a CT of the thorax showing a 1.9cm x 3.9cm enhancing anterior mediastinal mass with an internal focus of calcification (arrow).

Figure 44.2 is a CT of the abdomen revealing dilatation of the jejunum with marked small bowel wall thickening.

What is your differential diagnosis?

- Infective.
- Neoplastic.
- Inflammatory (the subacute onset of symptoms, fever and very high CRP in this age group is atypical for inflammatory bowel disease).

What would you do next?

In view of the CT findings, an oesophagogastroduodenoscopy/push enteroscopy is arranged for endoscopic correlation (Figure 44.3) and to obtain histology to guide management (Figure 44.4-44.6).

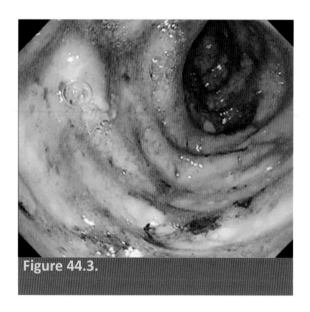

Figure 44.3.

Please describe what you see

Figure 44.3 shows diffuse inflammatory exudates and friable mucosa extending from the distal oesophagus down to the 4th part of the duodenum and beyond. Biopsies are taken.

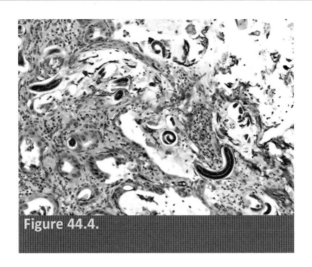

Figure 44.4.

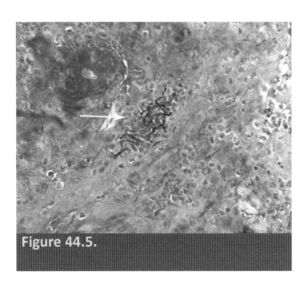

Figure 44.5.

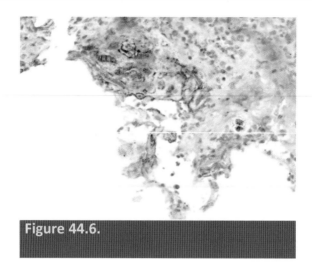

Figure 44.6.

Please describe what you see

Biopsies reveal *Strongyloides filariform* larvae in the stomach and duodenum (Figure 44.4). Fungal spores are present on periodic acid-Schiff staining (Figure 44.5), and *Herpes simplex* virus immunohistochemistry is also positive from the oesophageal biopsy (Figure 44.6).

How would you treat this patient?

He is started on ivermectin (antiparasitic), micafungin (antifungal) and valganciclovir (antiviral). However, he subsequently develops respiratory failure requiring intensive care unit admission with subsequent bronchoalveolar lavage also showing *Strongyloides* larvae.

Clinical pearls

- *Strongyloides stercoralis* can undergo a unique auto-infective lifecycle whereby it can reproduce entirely within the human host.
- It is found globally and is endemic to rural tropical and subtropical Southeast Asia.

- Manifestations of infection can range from subclinical in immunocompetent individuals to the highly fatal hyperinfection syndrome (HS) and disseminated disease in the immunocompromised host.
- The risk factors for hyperinfection syndrome occur in the immunocompromised patient [1]:
  - prolonged courses of high-dose steroids;
  - cytotoxic drugs;
  - anti-TNF therapy;
  - haematopoietic stem cell transplantation;
  - human T-lymphotropic virus type I (HTLV-I) infection;
  - human immunodeficiency virus (HIV) infection;
  - underlying malignancy;
  - hypogammaglobulinaemia (myeloma, combined variable immunodeficiency, etc.);
  - congenital immunodeficiency.

Treatment options for strongyloidiasis are [2]:

- Albendazole.
- Thiabendazole.
- Ivermectin (best option for an immunocompromised host).

Impress your attending

What would be a possible cause for this patient's immunosuppressed state?

An enhancing anterior mediastinal mass with calcification is noted on the CT. This raises the suspicion for Good's syndrome.

What is Good's syndrome?

Good's syndrome (thymoma with immunodeficiency) is a rare primary immunodeficiency in adults characterised by hypogammaglobulinaemia with B- and T-cell deficiency, which increases the susceptibility to infections such as encapsulated bacteria and other opportunistic organisms [3].

How would you minimise the risk of recurrent infection?
Referral to cardiothoracic surgery for consideration of surgical removal or debulking of the tumour. For this patient, an elective thymectomy is subsequently performed which confirms the diagnosis of a thymoma (type AB). He is currently on monthly intravenous immunoglobulin infusions to maintain adequate trough IgG values.

References

1. Corti M. *Strongyloides stercoralis* in immunosuppressed patients. *Arch Clin Infect Dis* 2016; 11(1): e27510.
2. Varatharajalu R, Rao KV. *Strongyloides stercoralis*: current perspectives. *Reports Parasitol* 2016; 5: 23-33.
3. Kelleher P, Misbah SA. What is Good's syndrome? Immunological abnormalities in patients with thymoma. *J Clin Pathol* 2003; 56: 12-6.

Case 45

History

A 55-year-old gentleman presents with epigastric discomfort which he has had for 2 years. He denies tarry stools, haematemesis, dysphagia or weight loss. He has a past history of hypertension and ischaemic heart disease. He is taking aspirin and nifedipine. He has had no previous endoscopic work-up.

Physical examination

- Temperature 37.1°C, pulse 72 bpm, BP 135/85mmHg, SaO$_2$ 98-100% on RA.
- Hydration is satisfactory.
- Examination of the hands reveals no clubbing and normal-appearing palmar creases.
- Head and neck examination is unremarkable.
- Cardiovascular: HS dual, no murmur.
- His chest is clear on auscultation.
- Abdominal examination reveals a soft, non-tender abdomen.
- No signs of oedema.

Investigations

- CBC:
  - WBC 5.9 x 10^9/L;
  - haemoglobin 12.5g/dL;
  - platelets 285 x 10^9/L.

What is your differential diagnosis of his epigastric discomfort?

- Peptic ulcer disease.
- Gastro-oesophageal reflux disease (GORD).
- Malignancy (e.g. liver, oesophageal, gastric).
- Pancreatic disease (chronic pancreatitis).
- Gastroparesis.
- Functional dyspepsia.

An oesophagogastroduodenoscopy (OGD) is performed showing the following (Figures 45.1 and 45.2).

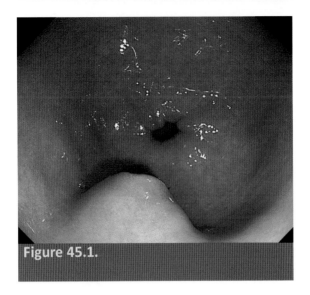

Figure 45.1.

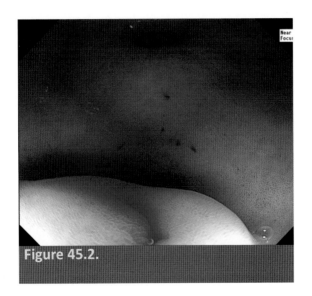

Figure 45.2.

Please describe what you see

The endoscopic photos show an antral submucosal nodule with an umbilicated appearance. The overlying mucosa appears normal.

What is the differential diagnosis?

- Ectopic pancreas.
- Carcinoid tumours.
- Lymphomas.
- Gastrointestinal stromal tumours (GISTs).

Which of the above is more likely, and why?

An ectopic pancreas.

The presence of the characteristic round shape and central depression makes an ectopic pancreas more likely.

How would you differentiate ectopic pancreas from the other differential diagnoses?

Radiological imaging, such as computed tomography (CT) and magnetic resonance imaging (MRI), provides information for the differential diagnosis of GI tumours, but they are limited in diagnosing small lesions within the gastric wall [1].

Endoscopic ultrasound (EUS) can assist in distinguishing these small subepithelial lesions [1].

What is the appearance of an ectopic pancreas on EUS?

The typical EUS features of an ectopic pancreas include heterogeneous echogenicity, indistinct borders and the presence of an anechoic area and location within the second, third, fourth and/or fifth layers [1-3].

What is the role of EUS-guided fine needle aspiration (FNA) or endoscopic removal of lesions in the diagnosis?

The diagnosis of an ectopic pancreas can be made if the typical endoscopic or endosonographic features are present.

EUS-guided FNA or endoscopic removal of the lesion may be considered if the typical endosonographic features of an ectopic pancreas cannot be well demonstrated [4].

The EUS shows the typical features of an ectopic pancreas. The patient remains asymptomatic.

How would you manage this patient?

For asymptomatic patients, no treatment is required [5].

For symptomatic patients, patients with complications or patients with diagnostic uncertainty, resection is advocated [5].

Resection can be done by surgery, endoscopic mucosal resection or endoscopic submucosal dissection [6, 7].

Clinical pearls

- An ectopic pancreas may present with a submucosal mass with a characteristic central depression.
- EUS may be helpful to differentiate an ectopic pancreas from other submucosal lesions of the gastrointestinal tract.
- An asymptomatic ectopic pancreas with characteristic imaging features may be observed.
- Resection should be considered in symptomatic patients, patients with complications and patients with diagnostic uncertainty.

Impress your attending

What is an ectopic pancreas?
An ectopic pancreas, also known as a pancreatic rest, is the presence of pancreatic tissue outside of its typical location without anatomic or vascular connections to the pancreas [8].

What are the common sites for an ectopic pancreas?
The common site of an ectopic pancreas is located in the GI tract: stomach (26%-38%), duodenum (28%-36%) and jejunum (16%) [9].

Lesions have also been reported in the colon, spleen, liver, Meckel's diverticulum, gallbladder, bile ducts, or fallopian tubes [10].

What are the possible complications of an ectopic pancreas?
Acute and chronic ectopic pancreatitis, pseudocyst, a palpable abdominal mass, gastrointestinal haemorrhage, gastric outlet obstruction and adenocarcinoma have all been reported [5].

References

1. Chou JW, Cheng KS, Ting CF, *et al*. Endosonographic features of histologically proven gastric ectopic pancreas. *Gastroenterol Res Pract* 2014; 2014: 160601.
2. Matsushita M, Hajiro K, Okazaki K, Takakuwa H. Gastric aberrant pancreas: EUS analysis in comparison with the histology. *Gastrointest Endosc* 1999; 49: 493-7.
3. Park SH, Kim GH, Park DY, *et al*. Endosonographic findings of gastric ectopic pancreas: a single center experience. *J Gastroenterol Hepatol* 2011; 26: 1441-6.
4. Chen SH, Huang WH, Feng CL, *et al*. Clinical analysis of ectopic pancreas with endoscopic ultrasonography: an experience in a medical center. *J Gastrointest Surg* 2008; 12(5): 877-81.
5. Attwell A, Sams S, Fukami N. Induction of acute ectopic pancreatitis by endoscopic ultrasound with fine-needle aspiration. *Clin Gastroenterol Hepatol* 2014; 12(7): 1196-8.

6. Khashab MA, Cummings OW, Dewitt JM. Ligation-assisted endoscopic mucosal resection of gastric heterotopic pancreas. *World J Gastroenterol* 2009; 15: 2805-8.

7. Ryu DY, Kim GH, Park DY, *et al.* Endoscopic removal of gastric ectopic pancreas: an initial experience with endoscopic submucosal dissection. *World J Gastroenterol* 2010; 16: 4589-93.

8. Armstrong CP, King PM, Dixon JM, Macleod IB. The clinical significance of heterotopic pancreas in the gastrointestinal tract. *Br J Surg* 1981; 68(6): 384-7.

9. O'Malley RB, Maturen KE, Al-Hawary MM, Mathur AK. Case of the season: ectopic pancreas. *Semin Roentgenol* 2013; 48(3): 188-91.

10. Lee MJ, Chang JH, Maeng H, *et al.* Ectopic pancreas bleeding in the jejunum revealed by capsule endoscopy. *Clin Endosc* 2012; 45(3): 194-7.

Case index

Index